PARKINSON'S DISEASE

100 MAXIMS

Volume 2 in the Series
100 Maxims in Neurology
Series Editor
Roger J. Porter MD

OTHER VOLUMES IN THE SERIES

PARKINSON'S DISEASE
100 MAXIMS

**John G. Nutt,
John P. Hammerstad and
Stephen T. Gancher**

*Department of Neurology,
Oregon Health Sciences University,
Portland, Oregon*

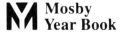
**Mosby
Year Book**

St. Louis Baltimore Boston Chicago London Philadelphia Sydney Toronto

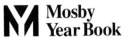
Mosby
Year Book
Dedicated to Publishing Excellence

© 1992 J. G. Nutt, J. P. Hammerstad and S. T. Gancher

First published in Great Britain 1992 by Edward Arnold,
a division of Hodder and Stoughton Limited

Published in the U.S. by Mosby-Year Book, Inc.
11830 Westline Industrial Drive
St. Louis, MO 63146

Whilst the advice and information in this book is believed to be true and accurate at the date of going to press, neither the author nor the publisher can accept any legal responsibility or liability for any errors or omissions that may be made. In particular (but without limiting the generality of the preceding disclaimer) every effort has been made to check drug dosages; however, it is still possible that errors have been missed. Furthermore, dosage schedules are constantly being revised and new side effects recognised. For these reasons the reader is strongly urged to consult the drug companies' printed instructions before administering any of the drugs recommended in this book.

Library of Congress Cataloging-in-Publication Data

Nutt, John G.
    Parkinson's disease / by John G. Nutt, J. P. Hammerstad,
  S. T. Gancher.
      p. cm.—(100 maxims in neurology)
    Includes index.
    ISBN 0-8016-7279-1
    1. Parkinsonism. I. Hammerstad, J. P. II. Gancher, S. T.
  III. Title. IV. Series.
    [DNLM: 1. Parkinson Disease—diagnosis. 2. Parkinson Disease—
  therapy. WL 359 N977p]
  RC382.N88 1992
  616.8'33—dc20
  DNLM/DLC
  for Library of Congress   92-49799
                                               CIP

Dedication

We dedicate this book to the many patients and professional colleagues who have shared with us their experiences in coping with parkinsonism and have thus shaped this book.

Acknowledgements

We thank Julie Carter, RN, ANP, for teaching us that management of Parkinson's disease is not just pharmacotherapy, the series editor, Roger Porter MD, for his editorial assistance, and Michelle Leaver for assembling multiple drafts into a finished manuscript.

Foreword to the 100 Maxims in Neurology Series

This second volume of the *100 Maxims* series follows quickly upon the first, and represents a special moment for all of us. These unique books in neurology derive from five years of patience, persistence and hard work.

The origin of the series lies in the early 1980s, when I began thinking about how a firm grasp of the fundamentals of diagnosis and treatment of epilepsy could benefit a physician confronted by this difficult disorder. In 1984, thanks to the generosity of Lord Walton of Detchant, my own book, *Epilepsy: 100 Elementary Principles*, was included in his prestigious series, *Major Problems in Neurology*. The second edition (W. B. Saunders) was published in 1989.

The real challenge, however, was to create an entire series on the notion that physicians like – insofar as is possible – to have concrete rules to guide their diagnosis and therapy. Even the best doctors, those with great knowledge and sensitive insight, lean on their experience of what has proven to be correct – and what has not. Thus was born the *100 Maxims in Neurology* series. The neurological disorders that we have chosen for this series lend themselves to 100 guiding principles for diagnosis and treatment. Discipline on the part of the authors has been necessary in order to reach, but not to exceed, this number. The books are intended to be monographs, although a few will combine the expertise of as many as three authors. Each book will be well referenced to make certain that the opinions expressed can be fortified by further reading.

The concept of '100 Maxims' is a specific service to the reader; each author is forced to unequivocally say what is important (and, by exclusion, what is less important). The ideal list of maxims comes from the author's own experience, as well as from recognition of those errors of diagnosis and treatment made most frequently. The format requires that the author be committed to a specific plan of action. Even though the text generally 'qualifies' the maxim, each maxim stands on its own as a declarative statement. Most textbooks are much less concrete in their recommendations regarding diagnosis and therapy. In summary, *100 Maxims* obliterates the curious dichotomy of the professor who is highly specific in verbal recommendations to students but enormously cautious in book chapters on the same subject!

I am grateful to many, but most especially to my wife, Candace, who has continuously supported my efforts, and to Editorial Staff of Edward Arnold Publishers, without whose encouragement and perseverance this series could not have been created.

Roger J Porter
1 February 1992

Foreword to this Volume

Parkinson's Disease: 100 Maxims is the second book in the *100 Maxims in Neurology* series. In this outstanding treatise, Drs Nutt, Hammerstad and Gancher address one of the most common yet clinically challenging disorders of the nervous system.

The authors start, in classical style, with diagnosis and its pitfalls. The reader is taught both the importance of an appropriate medical history and the nuances of subtle and insidious physical signs. The emphasis on physician as observer – rather than as evaluator of tests – is a healthy corrective in these times of passion for instrumentation. The sections on therapy are logical and precise; tips for the beneficial and appropriate use of the many medications abound. Few doctors who treat patients with Parkinson's disease will fail to profit from the experience cited here. But the book is not limited to doctors and drugs; the authors comprehensively explore the other avenues required to ameliorate the lives of those suffering from parkinsonism.

Drs Nutt, Hammerstad and Gancher have elucidated the most important principles of diagnosis and therapy in this complex disorder. True to the *100 Maxims* series, they have confined themselves to the 100 that are most important. Their experience and special expertise in Parkinson's disease is already well recognized, but now, in this book, we profit from their careful exposition on the complete care of the afflicted patient. I commend this volume to all who treat patients with this disorder.

Roger J Porter
1 February 1992

Preface

Parkinson's disease is common. Most physicians caring for adults will have patients with parkinsonism in their practice. The care of patients with parkinsonism is complex. At the time of diagnosis, the patient may only need education about the disease and reassurance. But over the ensuing years, the physician may be orchestrating pharmacologic interventions, other medical consultations, and a variety of community and medical services to cope with a diversity of problems that may be associated with parkinsonism.

There are a number of excellent monographs on parkinsonism and movement disorders. However, they tend to be medical compendiums of what is known about the disorder rather than guides to diagnosis and management. In this work, we have attempted to extract the information that is essential for managing patients with parkinsonism and to put it into the context of our experience in caring for these patients. Optimal care of parkinsonian patients requires more than just intelligent use of antiparkinsonian drugs and we have detailed these other, often less appreciated, aspects of management. We will be very satisfied if this work helps physicians offer better care to people with parkinsonism.

Contents

Chapter 4 Diagnosis: What is the Cause of the Parkinsonism?

Chapter 9 Therapy: Levodopa in Later Stages of the Disease

Chapter 10 Therapy: Dopamine Agonists

Chapter 11 Non-Pharmacological Interventions

Chapter 12 Affective, Cognitive and Sleep Disturbances

Chapter 13 Autonomic and Vegetative Functions

Chapter 14 Special Considerations

Chapter 15 Future Therapies

Index   163

1
Introduction and Epidemiology

1. Every physician should be familiar with parkinsonism

Parkinsonism is a common disorder. Between 1 and 2 persons per 1000 of the Caucasian population are estimated to have parkinsonism (Martilla, 1987). Men are affected slightly more commonly than women. The disorder begins in later life with an average age of onset of 60. The incidence of the disorder increases with age, leading to the suggestion that everyone would develop parkinsonism if they lived long enough. Because of the late onset of the illness, the prevalence increases to 1 in 100 if one looks at the population that is older than 55 years of age. For this reason, regardless of specialty, most physicians caring for adult patients will be treating individuals with parkinsonism.

The presentation may be subtle; early symptoms are often interpreted as aging, musculoskeletal problems or other systemic illnesses for which the patient may consult a variety of physicians. And, in fact, the initial diagnosis of parkinsonism is most often made, or at least suspected, by a non-neurologist and later confirmed by a neurologist. Not only recognizing early parkinsonism, but separating parkinsonism from other degenerative disorders or determining its etiology, may at times be a diagnostic challenge.

The therapy of parkinsonism is challenging yet rewarding because most patients are moderately to markedly improved by therapy. Furthermore, many drugs used for other medical purposes can induce parkinsonism or interact with antiparkinsonian agents. For these reasons all physicians need some familiarity with the principles of therapy for parkinsonism. As the disease progresses, a variety of side-effects and late manifestations of the disorder may complicate therapy and tax the ingenuity of the primary physician and consultants.

2.   *Prepare for an enduring relationship with the parkinsonian patient*

Parkinsonism is a chronic progressive disorder. The life expectancy of a patient with the disease now approaches that of the normal population, a change brought about by the introduction of levodopa (Martilla, 1987). This means that the average patient will be followed for 15 years. During that time the patient's disability will progress, requiring modifications of therapy and continuing support and education.

The rate of progression of parkinsonism is variable. In some patients the disease progresses slowly for many years, being more of 'a damned nuisance' rather than a disability. For these patients, tremor, rather than bradykinesia, is the dominant feature. In other patients the disease is more aggressive with significant disability appearing within a few years of onset. Patients with 'parkinsonism plus' syndromes, to be discussed later, or with predominant rigidity and axial signs such as dysarthria and postural instability, do less well.

Reference

Martilla RJ. Epidemiology. In: Koller WC (ed), *Handbook of Parkinson's Disease*. New York: Marcel Dekker, 1987: 35–50.

2
Diagnosis: Is it Parkinsonism? – Major Symptoms and Signs of the Disorder

3. *Parkinsonism is a syndrome characterized by tremor, rigidity, bradykinesia and postural disturbances*

Parkinsonism is a constellation of signs that constitute a syndrome with multiple etiologies. Clinically, Parkinson's disease is often used to designate parkinsonism that is idiopathic. Pathologically, Parkinson's disease usually implies the presence of the neuronal cytoplasmic inclusions, Lewy bodies, in the remaining dopaminergic neurons and other deep nuclei, in a patient with a clinical diagnosis of parkinsonism. The definition of Parkinson's disease, clinically and pathologically, is under scrutiny, but the concept of parkinsonism as a syndrome is not.

Parkinsonism is defined solely by clinical signs. The diagnosis of parkinsonism is dependent upon the physician's assessment of the history and the presence of tremor, rigidity, bradykinesia and postural disturbances. Two or more of these four cardinal signs of parkinsonism should be present. There are no laboratory tests that confirm or refute the clinical diagnosis. Laboratory tests do provide possible etiologies for the syndrome.

A not uncommon problem is the patient who presents with the diagnosis of parkinsonism and is receiving antiparkinsonian medications but in whom the history of the exam makes the physician uncertain of the diagnosis. In this situation, the withdrawal of drugs may clarify the issue. It is important to realize that emergence of parkinsonism may take days to weeks after discontinuing the antiparkinsonian agents. Tapering the drugs avoids precipitous worsening.

4. *Parkinsonism presents with an insidious development of impaired handwriting and difficulty rolling over in bed*

The onset is gradual and therefore often escapes the patient's and patient's family's recognition. Frequently, a friend or relative who has not seen the patient in months or years suddenly calls attention to the decline in motor function. Alternatively, the presence of the signs of parkinsonism may be brought to the patient's attention by new situations that demand normal motor control or by stressful situations that bring out tremor and highlight motor impairments. Careful questioning of the patient and family will reveal changes in speech and facial expression, arm swing, speed of walking and performance of the activities of daily living that preceded the patient's recognition of parkinsonism by months or years. A truly sudden – or even very rapid – onset of the signs should make the physician question the diagnosis or look particularly hard for an etiology of the parkinsonism.

Table 4.1 Common symptoms and signs of early parkinsonism

Facies	Less play of facial expression
Speech	Less distinct, softer
Fine motor tasks	Difficulties with handwriting, using hand tools and kitchen utensils, grooming, doing and undoing buttons
Postural	Difficulty rolling in bed and getting out of chairs or automobiles
Gait	Slowing, dragging one foot, loss of arm swing
Sensory	Stiffness and discomfort in an arm

5. *All that shakes is not necessarily parkinsonism*

Tremors are rhythmical oscillatory movements that are categorized by the activities and positions which maximize the motion. Action (intention) tremor is most prominent with active movement – for example, on finger to nose testing – and is generally indicative of cerebellar dysfunction. Postural tremor is most evident with a sustained posture and is most frequently reported by the patient as interfering with drinking from a cup. Resting tremor is tremor that is maximal when the body part is not in use; it often occurs when the hand is lying in the lap or hanging by the side and disappears when the limb is employed in purposeful activities. Because of this latter feature of resting tremor, it rarely causes much disability but is a cosmetic concern or simply a 'damned nuisance'. Resting tremor usually has a frequency of 4–6 cycles per second, slower than other forms of tremor.

Resting tremor is characteristic of parkinsonism and, in fact, resting tremor is almost pathognomonic of basal ganglia disorders. Tremor is the sign most commonly leading to the diagnosis of parkinsonism. In a series of 34 autopsy-proven cases of idiopathic parkinsonism, all had rest tremor, although in a third of the cases it was inconspicuous (Rajput, 1991). Patients with parkinsonism but no rest tremor often have 'parkinsonism plus' syndromes (Rajput, 1991). Between 40 and 50% of patients have postural and action tremors as well as resting tremor (Lance, 1963).

Resting tremor characteristically begins on one side of the body, most commonly in the hand, and then may spread, over months or years, to the other ipsilateral limb and then to the other side of the body and perhaps the cranial musculature (particularly mentalis, jaw and tongue muscles). It may remain asymmetrical through the course of the disorder. Resting tremor is exacerbated by stress and fatigue, as are other types of tremor. Tremor, particularly in mildly affected patients, is frequently present intermittently and should be looked for when the patient is stressed during the history-taking and exam. Mental status testing often brings it out. Watching the patient write and drink from a cup are helpful in distinguishing resting tremor from other tremor. The patient with parkinsonism and resting tremor will have small, irregular and laborious handwriting; the patient with postural tremor has large, tremulous writing. The patient with resting tremor will have no difficulty drinking from a cup but this task will be difficult for the patient with postural tremor. The parkinsonian patient with postural tremor, either alone or in combination with a rest tremor, may have other features of essential tremor, including a family history of tremor and amelioration of the tremor by alcohol. The critical point, however, is to avoid diagnosing parkinsonism based only on tremor; the patient must have rigidity and bradykinesia as well. Cogwheeling is not essential for the diagnosis of parkinsonism, and a ratchety resistance to passive movement of the limb may be felt by the examiner in patients who have other types of tremor and do not have rigidity. Cogwheeling may be a useful sign when elicited in a patient with rigidity and no observable tremor; in that setting the sign suggests the diagnosis of parkinsonism.

Table 5.1   Etiologies of postural tremors

Drugs	Lithium, tricyclics, steroids, adrenergic agonists, valproate, methylxanthines
Metabolic	Hyperthyroidism, Wilson's disease, metabolic encephalopathies, alcohol and drug withdrawal
Familial	Essential tremor
Other neurologic disorders	Peripheral neuropathy, focal and generalized dystonias, miscellaneous extrapyramidal disorders, Friedreich's ataxia

The entity most commonly mistaken for parkinsonism is essential tremor. This is a common disorder of adults, generally inherited as an autosomal dominant trait and presenting as an alcohol responsive postural tremor affecting head, voice and upper limbs. Legs are infrequently affected – the tremor tends to be more symmetrical than resting tremor. Other parkinsonian features are absent. Postural tremor, unlike rest and action tremors, has a long differential (Table 5.1).

6. *Akinesia and bradykinesia are best detected by casual observation*

Akinesia, absence or poverty of movement, is commonly manifested by reduced blink rate, decreased emotional play of facial muscles, paucity of fidgety or repositioning movements, decreased tendency either to cross the legs when sitting or to gesture with the hands while talking, and reduced associated movements such as swinging the arms while walking. Bradykinesia, slowness of movement, is often apparent when the patient undresses, searches his pockets or her purse, or enters and exits the examining room. Bradykinesia is not a fixed neurologic sign. The speed with which the patient carries out a motor act is influenced by the patient's motivation. Hence the patient may exhibit little bradykinesia during the formal neurologic exam even though slowness of movement is evident when the patient is not aware of being observed. The extreme example of the changeableness of bradykinesia is paradoxical kinesis, in which chair-bound or bed-bound parkinsonian patients are briefly capable of normal motor responses under duress – such as the home catching fire.

Difficulties with maintaining the timing and magnitude of repetitive motor acts is a common sign in parkinsonism. A particularly sensitive indicator of this abnormality is tapping the tip of the index finger on the distal interphalangeal joint of the thumb. The parkinsonian patient will have difficulty sustaining a rhythm and will tend to slow down or to have arrests of the tapping followed by speeding up of the tapping. Although the magnitude of each tap will vary, a tendency for each tap to become smaller is frequently observed. Watching the patient write will reveal the same motor disturbances – an inability to maintain a smooth flow of the pen and a progressive shrinking of the size of the letters. Tapping the heel on the floor is another motor task that discloses difficulties with motor timing. Surprisingly, the standard neurologic test of rapid alternating movements of the hands is less sensitive than the motor tasks above.

There are two caveats. First, difficulty with repetitive movements is not pathognomonic of parkinsonism; other motor lesions may also cause the same disturbances. Even micrographia, thought to be a classical sign of parkinsonism, may be produced by parietal lesions. Second, sometimes parkinsonism may present with an increased blink rate or with increased fidgety movements because the patient has akathisia (see maxim 90).

7. *Watching the patient arise from a chair, walk, and recover from postural perturbations detects deficits in postural reflexes*

Postural disturbances of parkinsonism may be classified as static or kinetic. Static postural abnormalities include scoliosis – often concave to the less affected side – and a flexed posture which gives the patient a stooped or simian appearance. Other static postural abnormalities include the tendency for the patient to stand with the knees slightly flexed and the elbows, wrists and metacarpal–phalangeal joints flexed, well illustrated by the drawing in Gowers' 1888 textbook (Fig. 7.1).

Kinetic postural disturbances often produce major disabilities. In bed, the patient may have difficulty organizing the limb and truncal movements

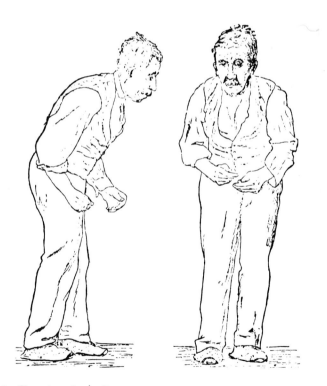

Fig. 7.1 Drawing from Gowers' 1888 text, *Diseases of the Nervous System*, illustrating the typical posture of moderately severe parkinsonism

to roll over, a surprisingly common complaint early in the course of parkinsonism. While sitting, the patient may tend to lean or drift slowly to one side or backwards. Upon attempting to stand, the patient may not appropriately move his feet under his center of mass and therefore have difficulty rising. When walking, turns are executed slowly and the trunk does not twist, producing the 'en bloc' appearance.

Postural stability is best tested with the examiner standing behind the patient and, after explaining the procedure, unexpectedly pulling the patient backwards by the shoulders. A normal person should resist this backwards displacement by one or two steps; the parkinsonian patient may require several steps or even start to fall. For this reason, the examiner must be prepared to catch the patient. Patients adapt to this test; therefore, the first pull is often the most revealing. Despite this evidence of postural instability, parkinsonian patients do not widen their base and may even be able to balance on one foot. In contrast, the patient with cerebellar dysfunction may be unable to stand on a narrow base but have an adequate, although dysmetric, response to postural perturbation.

8. Increased tone may be difficult to interpret

An increase in resistance to passive movement of limb joints is characteristic of parkinsonism. This rigidity has a plastic or lead-pipe quality; the increased tone is present throughout the range of motion of the joint and is not sensitive to the speed with which the limb is moved. It is most sensitively detected at the patient's wrist and elbow while the examiner slowly and in an unpredictable manner moves both joints simultaneously. Rigidity in the trunk and shoulders may be detected by grasping the standing patient by the shoulders near the base of the neck and gently rotating the trunk to assess both the resistance to the movement and the arm swing. Some rigidity of the neck is a common sign in the elderly, and must be interpreted with caution. Rigidity in the legs is also often difficult to assess accurately; patients simply cannot relax the legs as well as the arms.

Rigidity can be augmented by having the patient draw a circle in the air with one arm while the examiner tests for rigidity in the other arm. The examiner may note a moderate to marked increase in the passive resistance to movement with this maneuver. Be careful! This effect is not unique to parkinsonism and may be seen in many healthy elderly individuals. However, this test may be useful to detect mild asymmetrical rigidity and sometimes will bring out cogwheeling that is not apparent without augmentation.

As rigidity is only one cause of increased muscle tone, the physician must try to differentiate rigidity, implicating basal ganglia disease, from other forms of increased tone. One problem commonly encountered is a patient who is unable to relax. In such patients the observation of arm swing while walking rapidly may be the most reliable manner in which to assess the presence of rigidity.

A second form of increased tone is spasticity, defined as a velocity-dependent resistance to passive movement. Thus, with very slow movement of the spastic limb, no resistance may be present; with rapid movement, a rapid rise in resistance is followed by a disappearance of the resistance, the so-called spastic catch. This velocity-dependence of the resistance is in contrast to rigidity in which the resistance is independent of the speed of passive movement and hence is characterized as plastic. Brisk deep tendon reflexes (DTRs) and Babinski signs are, of course, suggestive of spasticity, but the DTRs tend to be brisker on the more parkinsonian side in the asymmetrically affected patient, an observation which can sometimes mislead the physician (see maxim 9). Spasticity is characteristic of corticospinal dysfunction.

The third type of increased tone is *gegenhalten* or paratonia, an uneven resistance to passive movement with the patient seemingly unconsciously resisting or aiding the examiner's attempts to move the limb. This tone abnormality is similar to that seen in patients who are unable to relax, but when severe is commonly associated with dementia and widespread neurological dysfunction. Increased tone may be a product of more than one of the above phenomena and the physician may be unable to separate out the pathology responsible for it.

Surprisingly, rigidity does not cause akinesia and bradykinesia. Most patients with rigidity do have bradykinesia and akinesia but patients may have severe akinesia without any trace of rigidity. In fact, there is a subset of parkinsonism termed pure akinesia without rigidity or tremor. Whether this group reflects a distinct syndrome is controversial (Quinn *et al.*, 1989). Another example of the disassociation of rigidity and bradykinesia is seen in patients who undergo thalamotomy. Rigidity and tremor is reduced but bradykinesia is not (maxim 94).

References

Gowers WR. *Disease of the Nervous System*. Philadelphia: F Blakiston, Son & Co., 1888.

Lance JW, Schwab RS, Peterson EA. Action tremor and the cogwheel phenomenon in Parkinson's disease. *Brain* 1963; **86**: 95–110.

Quinn NP, Luthert P, Honavar M, Marsden CD. Pure akainesia due to Lewy body Parkinson's disease: a case with pathology. *Mov Dis* 1989; **4**: 85–9.

Rajput AH, Rozdilsky B, Ang L. Occurrence of resting tremor in Parkinson's disease. *Neurology* 1991; **41** 1298–9.

3
Diagnosis: Less Common Features and Pitfalls

9. *Parkinsonism often begins on one side of the body and may be confused with hemiparesis*

In the majority of cases, the symptoms and signs of parkinsonism begin on one side of the body – usually the arm, followed by the leg on the same side. Although the other limbs eventually become symptomatic, this asymmetry may persist throughout the course of the disease, and is believed to reflect an asymmetrical loss of dopamine neurons in the substantia nigra.

This unilateral onset, particularly if not accompanied by tremor, can produce the false impression of a hemiparesis caused by some other slowly progressive disease, such as a brain tumor.

> A 48-year-old woman was admitted to hospital for investigation of a six-month history of weakness and clumsiness and paresthesias of the right arm. She was found to have a right facial droop, increased tone and decreased swing of the right arm, right reflex preponderance and a 'Babinski sign'. Because of a history of fluctuating symptoms she was investigated for multiple sclerosis. CSF, CT scan and VER were normal. Six months later the right 'hemiparesis' had progressed, and a CT scan was repeated to look for a brain tumor. Over the next twelve months she developed micrographia and more obvious rigidity of the right limbs. A trial of levodopa plus decarboxylase inhibitor (DCI) completely alleviated her 'hemiparesis'.

Bradykinesia and rigidity are often interpreted and described by the patient as weakness. The examiner may be misled by a slowing in voluntary contraction of muscles when testing motor power that is a result of parkinsonian bradykinesia but simulates weakness. Clumsiness and slowing of fine motor movements or repetitive movements such as finger tapping are indistinguishable from those produced by corticospinal lesions. Extrapyramidal rigidity may be misinterpreted as spasticity. An incomplete elevation and mild flexion of the arm when testing for pronator drift, a flexion posture of the arm and reduced arm swing, or a lag in the step and dragging of the foot also promote the impression of a hemiparesis. Occasionally there is a unilateral decrease in facial expression and mobility (hypomimea) on the same side mimicking a central facial paresis, and adding to the confusion. In some cases the tendon jerks are asymmetric and exaggerated on the symptomatic side. Finally, a persistent extension of the great toe ('striatal toe') can simulate a Babinski sign (for further discussion see maxim 24).

Careful attention to certain features of the exam can help differentiate unilateral parkinsonism from hemiparesis. A true Babinski sign is not present in idiopathic parkinsonism; even the tonically extended great toe ('striatal toe') will show the normal flexor response with plantar stimulation, distinguishing this nigrostriatal syndrome from a corticospinal lesion. The patient's increased tone has the characteristics of rigidity and not of spasticity (maxim 8). The presence of cogwheeling can further confirm the true nature of the increased tone. Look carefully for evidence of rigidity and bradykinesia in the other limbs. However, do not be misled by a mild increase in tone with contralateral activation, which is often present in normal elderly adults. A soft voice and facial masking with decreased blinking can suggest the right diagnosis. A flexed standing posture may provide a helpful clue that this is hemiparkinsonism rather than hemiparesis.

10.   *Pain and sensory symptoms can occur in parkinsonism*

Although the recognized pathology of parkinsonism primarily affects motor systems, approximately 40% of patients report primary sensory symptoms when specifically queried (Snider *et al.*, 1976; Koller, 1984). In contrast, only 8% of a control population report similar symptoms. Pain, numbness, and tingling paresthesias occur with about equal frequency, while burning or cold sensations are reported less often. In one study primary sensory symptoms preceded the onset of motor disability in 9% of patients, thereby complicating early diagnosis (Snider *et al.*, 1976). The symptoms usually occur on the side on which the motor symptoms first appear. The primary pain and sensory symptoms of idiopathic parkinsonism are not accompanied by any objective abnormalities on clinical exam; also, nerve conduction velocities and somatosensory evoked potentials are normal. Generally, a careful examination reveals bradykinesia or changes in tone in the painful limb. The most direct and efficient way to establish the source of the sensory symptoms and to avoid unnecessary testing is to place the patient on carbidopa/lerodopa (Sinemet) or a dopamine agonist; these medications almost invariably relieve the pain or paresthesias if they are caused by the parkinsonism.

A 56-year-old woman developed disagreeable cold and pulling sensations in her right arm and leg. She wore an extra stocking and a glove to warm her cold and numb foot and hand, which also tingled on occasion. Sometimes her right thigh felt hot while the rest of her limb was cold. When she developed 'stiffness' in her right leg she was investigated for a rheumatological condition. Nerve conduction studies and a lumbar CT scan were negative. The more she complained about the odd sensations the more convinced her doctors became that they were psychophysiologic. One year later a resting tremor appeared in her right foot. She was started on Sinemet and the sensory symptoms, stiffness and tremor were immediately alleviated.

Olfactory dysfunction is the only demonstrable sensory deficit found in parkinsonian patients. A recent study showed that 90% of patients had lower test scores on odor identification than their matched controls and 38% had severe dysfunction and were symptomatic (Doty *et al.*, 1988). The degree of dysfunction was unrelated to the severity or duration of disease. It is not specific to parkinsonism; olfaction is also impaired in Alzheimer's disease.

11.   *Parkinsonism commonly presents as a musculoskeletal disorder*

Rigidity and bradykinesia without tremor in an upper limb – described as a deep aching pain and stiffness – is a relatively common mode of onset of parkinsonism. Often the patient localizes the symptoms to the shoulder, giving the impression of a musculoskeletal disorder in that joint. In some instances, reduced mobility of the arm from bradykinesia leads to demonstrable shoulder pathology. In a survey of 150 patients and 60 matched controls, a significantly higher incidence of both a history of shoulder complaints (43% versus 23%) and frozen shoulder (12.7% versus 1.7%) was found in the parkinsonian population (Riley *et al.*, 1989). In at least 8% of the patients, frozen shoulder was the first symptom of disease, occurring up to two years prior to the onset of the more commonly recognized features of parkinsonism. Edema may occur in the hand, giving rise to a 'shoulder–hand syndrome'. Presumably the edema is due to stasis since it disappears when the extremity is mobilized by treatment with Sinemet or dopamine agonists.

The clues leading to the correct diagnosis are clumsiness and slowing of hand and finger or foot movements, micrographia, rigidity throughout the limb, cogwheeling, and the eventual appearance of tremor. Treatment is straightforward: relief of the bradykinesia with dopaminergic agents and mobilization of the shoulder with physical therapy.

The same approach applies to complaints of aching and stiffness in other body regions, neck, back and legs. If the musculoskeletal complaints arise from parkinsonian bradykinesia and rigidity, pharmacotherapy will relieve the complaints and avoid a needless search for other causes.

12.   *Hypophonia is common but dysarthria is unusual in early parkinsonism*

A decrease in the volume of the voice (hypophonia) is usually first noted by the spouse, who complains that the patient is mumbling, while the patient is equally convinced the spouse has a hearing problem. If the disagreement becomes sufficiently heated, the patient will win the argument in the early stages, because with emotion or voluntary effort the volume can be raised to normal levels. With time, however, the hypophonia becomes more difficult to overcome, and the patient may become just as frustrated as the spouse with this obstacle in communication. In addition to the decrease in volume the voice loses normal modulation and becomes more monotonal. The hypophonia probably results from bradykinesia and rigidity of respiratory muscles and is generally worse when the patient is tired or anxious.

More than a hundred muscles are involved in speech, producing phonemes at a rate of 14 per second (Critchley, 1981). In parkinsonism, as the orofacial and lingual bradykinesia rigidity worsen in the mid to later stages of the disease, phonemes are less well articulated, producing a hypokinetic dysarthria. A form of stuttering may occur in which the patient gets stuck on the first word of a phrase and repeats it several times. This palilalia often is associated with slurring of words together with speeding up towards the end of the sentence; it resembles the same phenomenon as in the gait, and is sometimes referred to as 'festinating speech'. Effective speech may be complicated further by respiratory difficulties secondary to levodopa-induced respiratory dyskinesia and dyspnea (maxim 85).

Dysarthria and dysphagia do not occur as prominent early symptoms in idiopathic parkinsonism; if present early in the course of the neurologic

Table 12.1   Abnormalities of voice and speech

Voice	Hypophonia
	Monotone pitch
	Change in quality – breathy, hoarse, higher pitched
Speech	Hesitation in starting and inappropriate silences
	Indistinct articulation of consonants
	Propulsive rushes (festination)
	Palilalia

Source: Darley *et al.* (1975)

disorder, other diagnoses should be considered, especially motor neuron disease, progressive supranuclear palsy, or multi-infarct state. Dysarthria associated with signs of a pseudobulbar palsy and pseudobulbar affect suggest these latter entities.

A disturbance in language function (aphasia) is not a feature of parkinsonism. Stroke, Alzheimer's disease or other disorders (which may have parkinsonian features) should be considered (see maxims 28, 29).

13.   *Jaw and tongue tremor are parkinsonism; head and voice tremor are essential tremor*

Like most dictums in medicine this rule is not absolute, but is a helpful guide in differentiating essential tremor from parkinsonism. In general, parkinsonian tremor is most common in the limbs, but sometimes is most prominent or occurs only in the head, jaw or tongue. Tremor confined to the head as a nodding 'yes' or 'no' tremor is rare in parkinsonism but is common as a variant of benign essential or familial tremor. Essential tremor of the jaw and/or tongue is almost invariably accompanied by a head tremor. Parkinsonian jaw and tongue tremor occur in the absence of head tremor and are usually accompanied by a typical resting tremor in the limbs.

Voice tremor never occurs in parkinsonism. In essential tremor, a tremorous voice is most often associated with a head tremor. Occasionally essential voice tremor occurs as an isolated problem; it may accompany spasmodic dysphonia, which also gives the voice a tight, strangulated quality.

14.   *Parkinsonism may simulate depression or aging*

Parkinsonism may be mistaken for the psychomotor retardation of depression, an understandable error because depression is relatively common in parkinsonism. Conversely, the psychomotor retardation of depression may mimic the bradykinesia and hypomimea of early parkinsonism. Distinguishing features suggestive of depression are the lack of tremor and rigidity and the presence of vegetative symptoms.

Differentiating the effects of normal aging on posture and gait from that of early parkinsonism can be challenging. Both produce a stooped posture and a slowing of gait. However, other features of parkinsonism are absent in the normal elderly person. In the latter, facial masking is seldom present. The typical resting tremor is also not present, although older persons commonly have a postural tremor ('senile tremor') which is sometimes mistaken for a parkinsonian tremor (see maxim 5). There is little, if any, increase in resting muscle tone. Slowing of movements occurs in aging; however, the pronounced fatigability that characterizes true bradykinesia is absent. True rigidity and bradykinesia in the extremities is absent in the normal aging person and freezing and a festinating gait are also not present.

References

Critchley EMR. Speech disorders of Parkinsonism: a review. *J Neurol Neurosurg Psychiat* 1981; **44**: 751–8.

Darley FL, Aronson AE, Brown JR. *Motor Speech Disorders*. Philadelphia: WB Saunders, 1975.

Doty RL, Deems DA, Stellar S. Olfactory dysfunction in parkinsonism: general deficit unrelated to neurologic signs, disease stage, or disease duration. *Neurology* 1988; **38**: 1237–44.

Koller WC. Sensory symptoms in Parkinson's disease. *Neurology* 1984; **34**: 957–9.

Riley D, Lang AE, Blair RDG, Birnbaum A, Reid B. Frozen shoulder and other shoulder disturbances in Parkinson's disease. *J Neurol Neurosurg Psychiat* 1989; **52**: 63–6.

Snider SR, Fahn S, Isgreen WP, Cote LJ. Primary sensory symptoms in parkinsonism. *Neurology* 1976; **26**: 423–9.

4
Diagnosis: What is the Cause of the Parkinsonism?

15. Parkinsonism is a syndrome, not a disease

The constellation of symptoms and signs we recognize as parkinsonism has many etiologies (Gibb, 1989a). Thus, once the physician has made a diagnosis of parkinsonism, the cause of the parkinsonism must be determined. Most commonly the syndrome is idiopathic, which traditionally has been designated as 'Parkinson's disease'. Some prefer to use the term 'idiopathic parkinsonism' to underscore that it is a syndrome with potentially multiple etiologies (Calne, 1989). The idiopathic form of parkinsonism is not a disease until we know the cause, just as we do not call ataxia 'ataxic disease' (Duvoisin, 1982).

Parkinsonism is caused by a dysfunction of dopaminergic neurotransmission in the nigrostriatal system or by lesions in the striatum or globus pallidus whose function is modulated by the nigrostriatal dopaminergic neurons. The anatomy and the neurotransmitters of the internal neuronal circuitry of the basal ganglia and the pathways that connect the basal ganglia with the other cerebral areas controlling movement (the motor, premotor, and supplementary motor cortices, thalamus and cerebellum) is summarized in Fig. 15.1 (Alexander and Crutcher, 1990). The main receiving station (for afferent input from the cerebral cortex) of the basal ganglia is the caudate/putamen (striatum) and the major transmitting stations (efferent output) are the medial globus pallidus and the zona reticulata of the substantia nigra (SNr), whose outputs are relayed to the supplementary motor cortex through the ventral thalamus. This loop from cortex through the basal ganglia back to the cortex allows the basal ganglia to modulate the motor output that ultimately is transmitted via the corticospinal system.

The output of the globus pallidus and the SNr is modulated by input received from the striatum via a direct and indirect pathway. The direct link is a GABAergic striatopallidal system that inhibits pallidal output neurons in the internal (medial) segment. The indirect pathway goes through the external (lateral) segment of the globus pallidus and the sub-

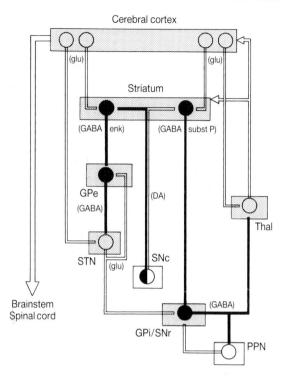

Fig. 15.1 Schematic diagram of the circuitry and neurotransmitters of the basal ganglia–thalamocortical circuitry, indicating the parallel 'direct' and 'indirect' pathways from the striatum to the basal ganglia output nuclei. Inhibitory neurons are shown as filled symbols, excitatory neurons as open symbols. *Abbreviations:* DA, dopamine; enk, enkephalin; GABA, gamma-aminobutyric acid; GPe, external segment of globus pallidus; GPi, internal segment of globus pallidus; glu, glutamate; PPN, pedunculopontine nucleus; SNc, substantia nigra pars compact; SNr, substantia nigra pars reticulata; subst P, substance P; STN, subthalamic nucleus; Thal, thalamus. (From Alexander and Crutcher, 1990)

thalamic nucleus. The loss of function in the nigrostriatal projection in idiopathic parkinsonism results in a decrease in striatal output in this system, disinhibiting the excitatory drive from the subthalamic neurons on the medial pallidal output neurons. This increase in pallidal activity is unopposed because of a reduction in striatal inhibitory drive via the direct pathway. The net result in parkinsonism is an increase in output from the medial globus pallidus which inhibits activity in the thalamocortical motor output (Fig. 15.2) (DeLong, 1990). Therefore, lesions or degeneration of any part of this neuronal circuitry – whose net effect is to increase pallidal outflow – may produce parkinsonism. Hence, potential etiologies of parkinsonism may be thought of as any biochemical process that interferes with dopaminergic neurotransmission or degenerative and structural lesions that result in excessive inhibition of the thalamocortical motor loop.

Examples of biochemical causes include pharmacologic agents that interfere with dopaminergic transmission, or toxins affecting the substantia nigra or globus pallidus. There are many degenerative or structural lesions affecting the striatum, globus pallidus or SN that can potentially cause parkinsonism (Table 15.1).

Although many of these causes of parkinsonism are rare, the physician should always search for treatable causes. Parkinsonism induced by dopamine antagonists (antipsychotic, antiemetic, antihypertensive drugs) that block the postsynaptic receptor in striatum are the most important to exclude because of its reversibility (see maxim 20). Most cases of secondary parkinsonism, however, turn out to be heterogenous system degenerations

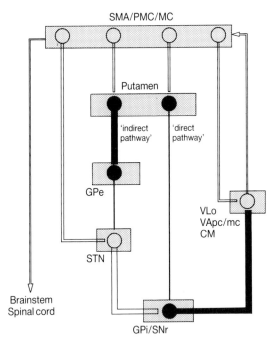

Fig. 15.2 Schematic representation of neuronal activity in the 'motor' circuit in parkinsonism. Excessive inhibition of GPe within the indirect pathway leads to disinhibition of the STN, which in turn provides excessive excitatory drive to the basal ganglia output nuclei (GPi/SNr), thus leading to excessive thalamic inhibition. This is reinforced by reduced inhibitory input to GPi/SNr through the direct pathway. Overall, these effects are postulated to result in a reduction in the usual reinforcing influence of the motor circuit upon cortically initiated movements. Inhibitory neurons are represented by filled symbols and excitatory neurons by open symbols. *Abbreviations:* CM, centromedian nucleus; GPe, external segment of the globus pallidus; GPi, internal segment of the globus pallidus; MC, primary motor cortex; PMC premotor cortex; SMA, supplementary motor area; SNr, substantia nigra pars reticulata; STN, subthalamic nucleus; VAmc, nucleus ventralis anterior pars magnocellularis; VApc, nucleus ventralis anterior pars parvocellularis; VLo, nucleus ventralis lateralis pars oralis. (From DeLong, 1990)

Table 15.1 Etiology of Parkinsonism

Pharmacologic	A. Drugs that interfere with DA synthesis, storage or release
	   1. alpha methylparatyrosine
	   2. reserpine
	   3. alpha methyldopa
	B. Drugs that block the DA receptor
	   1. antipsychotics
	   2. antihypertensive (Ca^{++} channel blockers)
	   3. antiemetic

Toxins	A. For substantia nigra
	   1. MPTP
	B. For globus pallidus
	   1. carbon monoxide
	   2. carbon disulfide
	   3. cyanide
	   4. manganese (also striatum)

Degenerations	A. Predominately DA neurons
	   1. idiopathic parkinsonism
	B. Heterogenous system degeneration of unknown cause—substantia nigra, striatum, pallidum and other neuronal systems ('parkinsonism-plus')
	   1. progressive supranuclear palsy (PSP)
	   2. multiple sytems atrophy
	   3. corticobasal degeneration
	   4. ALS/PD/dementia complex of Guam
	   5. diffuse Lewy body disease
	   6. Alzheimer's disease
	   7. Pick's disease
	C. Hereditary
	   1. Wilson's disease
	   2. Huntington's disease
	   3. spinocerebellar degenerations
	   4. Hallervorden–Spatz disease
	   5. familial parkinsonism
	   6. dopa-responsive dystonia with parkinsonism

Metabolic	A. Hypoparathyroidism B. Chronic hepatocerebral degeneration C. Calcification of the basal ganglia D. Leigh's disease E. Central pontine myelinolysis

Infectious transmissible	A. Encephalitis
	   1. encephalitis lethargica
	   2. AIDS
	   3. other encephalitides
	B. Creutzfeldt–Jakob disease
	C. Syphilis

Table 15.1   Etiology of Parkinsonism *(contd.)*

Structural lesions	A. Vascular (multi-infarct gait disorder) B. Normal-pressure hydrocephalus C. Tumor D. Trauma

in which the postsynaptic striatal neuron of the nigrostriatal dopaminergic circuit is diseased, with a reduction in striatal output to the medial pallidal neurons just as in idiopathic parkinsonism. Unlike idiopathic parkinsonism, however, the striatal neurons in these multisystem degenerations (e.g. PSP) are incapable of responding to dopaminergic stimulation, thus accounting for the poor response to levodopa or dopamine agonists.

16.   *Idiopathic parkinsonism is characterized by the Lewy body and striatal dopamine depletion*

About 85% of cases of parkinsonism are idiopathic. The pathologic hallmark of idiopathic parkinsonism is currently considered to be the degeneration of neurons in the substantia nigra pars compacta (especially the caudal central cell groups) whose axons terminate in the caudate and putamen (striatum) and release dopamine as their synaptic neurotransmitter (Fig. 16.1) (Jellinger, 1987). Experience with the neurotoxin MPTP which produces selective degeneration of neurons of the pars compacta (see maxim 21) indicates that the degeneration of these dopaminergic nigral neurons can account for all the motor manifestations of parkinsonism. Neuronal degeneration occurs less consistently and severely in other areas of the central nervous system and accounts for other features associated with idiopathic parkinsonism (Jellinger, 1987; Halliday *et al.*, 1990). Autonomic dysfunction is probably secondary to degeneration of neurons in the hypothalamus, dorsal motor nucleus of the vagus and sympathetic ganglia. Loss of the pigmented noradrenergic neurons in locus ceruleus could also contribute to autonomic dysfunction, as well as to disturbances of sleep and mentation. Involvement of the cholinergic neurons of the substantia innominata (including the nucleus basalis of Meynert) may be responsible for the cognitive changes in some parkinsonian patients.

The most characteristic pathologic marker of idiopathic parkinsonism is the Lewy body, an eosinophilic cytoplasmic inclusion body found in the neurons still remaining in the affected nuclei. Some authors require the presence of Lewy bodies in the substantia nigra to make the pathological diagnosis of idiopathic parkinsonism (Gibb and Lees, 1988). On the other hand, Lewy bodies are not entirely specific for idiopathic parkinsonism.

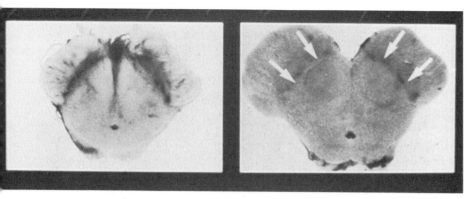

Fig. 16.1 Comparison of sections of midbrain from a normal brain (left) and from a patient with Parkinson's disease, illustrating the loss of neurons and depigmentation of substantia nigra in the parkinsonian brain.

Lewy bodies have been seen in brains of persons without parkinsonism (possibly presymptomatic parkinsonism?), in Alzheimer's disease, in the cortex of patients with severe dementia preceding parkinsonism ('cortical Lewy body disease'), and in anterior horn cells in motor neuron disease (Gibb and Lees, 1988). Thus, the Lewy body may be a nonspecific morphologic hallmark of cell death in a variety of neurodegenerative diseases.

Idiopathic parkinsonism can be thought of as a dopamine deficiency syndrome. The degeneration of the nigral dopaminergic neurons results in an 80–95% reduction in the content of dopamine in parkinsonian motor striatum (Bernheimer et al., 1973). This reduction in dopamine metabolism can be dramatically demonstrated with a PET scan of fluorodopa uptake in the striatum of patients with parkinsonism and in presymptomatic patients exposed to MPTP (Fig. 16.2). The fact that an 80% or greater loss of dopaminergic function is required for symptoms to appear indicates a remarkable ability of the system to compensate. Studies in experimental parkinsonism suggest several compensatory mechanisms are at work (Zigmond et al., 1990). Initially, normal extracellular concentrations of dopamine are maintained by increased activity and dopamine output by the surviving neurons (Robinson and Whishaw, 1988) and by reduction of the reuptake sites responsible for the removal of dopamine from the synaptic cleft (Zigmond et al., 1990). Later, as the synaptic concentration of dopamine falls, the postsynaptic receptors increase in number to increase the probability of an interaction with dopamine leading to a physiologic response (receptor supersensitivity). Finally, the degeneration of the dopamine neurons exceeds the capacity of these compensatory mechanisms and the symptoms appear. Both the concentration of dopamine and motor function can be restored by increasing the synthesis of dopamine by providing levodopa, the amino acid precursor of dopamine; another piece of evidence that the syndrome represents dopamine deficiency.

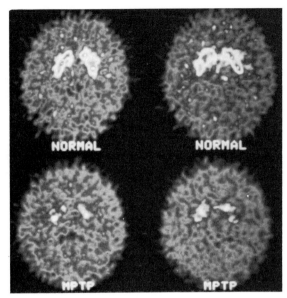

Fig. 16.2 PET scans after 6-fluorodopa administration in normals, a patient with PD and a presymptomatic individual exposed to MPTP. (From Calne, Langston, Martin *et al.*, 1985)

17.   *The genetic contribution to idiopathic parkinsonism is controversial*

Proposals as to the pathogenesis of the neuronal degeneration in idiopathic parkinsonism can be divided into genetic and environmental hypotheses (Table 17.1).

Common experience weighs against Mendelian inheritance as a common cause of idiopathic parkinsonism. However, cases of familial parkinsonism are regularly encountered (Golbe, 1990), leading to the suggestion that genetic factors may be responsible for some cases (Johnson, 1991). Several surveys, starting with Gowers, have noted that about 15% of parkinsonian patients have an affected relative. However, a lifetime incidence rate of 2.5% would be sufficient to account for this number by chance alone, and Duvoisin found equal prevalence of parkinsonism in the immediate family of patients as in the spouse's family (Duvoisin, 1982). Parkinsonism may be similar to Alzheimer's and ALS in which about 15% of the cases appear to be inherited and the remainder are sporadic.

Another approach to studying a Mendelian genetic contribution is the study of twins. However, three studies of monozygotic and dizygotic twins have failed to find a concordance rate that would support heredity as an important component (Ward *et al.*, 1983; Marttila *et al.*, 1988; Marsden, 1987). This conclusion is being challenged because of the possibility that

Table 17.1 Possible mechanisms in the pathogenesis of idiopathic parkinsonism

Genetic	A. Mendelian inheritance
	1. autosomal dominant
	2. multiple genes
	B. Defect in mitochondrial genome
Environmental	A. Viral
	B. Toxins
	1. industrial
	2. agricultural
	3. natural toxins in food
Interaction of environment and genetics	A. Defective detoxification of environmental toxins
	B. Increased generation or defective removal of free radicals

the incidence in the co-twins was underestimated (Johnson et al., 1990; Golbe, 1990). Some twin pairs were excluded from the analysis because one or both of them had 'atypical' features. This exclusion may have been inappropriate since idiopathic parkinsonism is not a well-defined nosologic entity; many cases are clinically atypical but with typical pathology. Another possible source of underestimation is a difference in age of onset. At the time of the study not enough time may have elapsed for the symptoms to appear in the co-twin. In the few concordant twin pairs identified, age at onset differed by 6.5 to 10 years. Affected members of a kindred with apparent autosomal dominant parkinsonism ranged in age of onset from 22 to 61 years. Positron emission tomographic studies of unaffected twins may yet reveal subclinical dopamine depletion and indicate a higher concordance rate than did the clinical examination.

Families have been reported in which two family members in different generations have developed parkinsonism almost simultaneously, leading to speculation that some familial cases may be due to a common exposure to an environmental toxin (Calne et al., 1987). The possibility that parkinsonism is caused by environmental factors acting on genetically susceptible individuals is attracting increasing attention. This merger of the genetic and environmental hypotheses is considered in maxim 19.

Patients often ask about the chances that their children will inherit the disease. This concern is sometimes triggered by knowledge of another affected member of the family. It is important not to accept this history at face value, especially if it is a second or third degree relative with whom the patient has little or no contact. Further investigation may reveal that the 'parkinsonism' is in fact a familial essential tremor or another disorder. Even if it is discovered to be parkinsonism, the parents still can be reassured that idiopathic parkinsonism is generally not inherited and that their offspring are not at much more risk for developing the disease than the general population.

18.   *Environmental factors are postulated to cause idiopathic parkinsonism*

Viruses were the first to receive serious attention as a possible cause of parkinsonism because of the epidemic of Von Economo's encephalitis from 1916 to 1926. Von Economo's encephalitis was notable for the frequency of parkinsonian features, although it seldom precisely mimicked idiopathic parkinsonism (Sacks, 1990). Oculomotor abnormalities and corticospinal signs were often present. Severe dysarthria and dysphagia were prominent. Paroxysms of tonic upward deviation of the eyes known as oculogyric crises were peculiar to this form of parkinsonism. A variety of respiratory abnormalities, tics and behavioral abnormalities were common (Duvoisin and Yahr, 1965). Encephalitis is now infrequently associated with parkinsonism (Rail, Scholte and Swash, 1981).

It has been proposed that cases of idiopathic parkinsonism appearing years later were due to a subclinical or latent infection. Because Von Economo's virus disappeared in 1926, the hypothesis predicted that new cases of idiopathic parkinsonism would not occur in individuals born after that year. Of course idiopathic parkinsonism has not disappeared and the incidence has not declined. The pathology of postencephalitic parkinsonism differs from that of idiopathic parkinsonism in that postencephalitic parkinsonism is characterized by neurofibrillary tangles and the absence of Lewy bodies (Hirano, 1970). Despite an extensive search, no virus – not even a 'slow virus' – has been implicated in the etiology of idiopathic parkinsonism.

Contemporary interest in environmental factors as the cause of idiopathic parkinsonism has been rekindled by developments on each side of the Pacific Ocean. One was the accidental discovery of the neurotoxin, 1-methyl-4-phenyl-1,2,3,6-tetrahydropyridine (MPTP) which was the unintentional byproduct of the synthesis of a meperidine analogue by clandestine laboratories. Injected by addicts, it produced signs typical of idiopathic parkinsonism (see maxim 21). The other development was the discovery of a high incidence of a neurodegenerative disease combining features of amyotrophic lateral sclerosis, parkinsonism, and dementia in the native Chamorro population of Guam. Epidemiologic evidence has excluded genetic and infectious causes and favors an environmental etiology for the neurologic syndrome (Spencer, 1987; Garruto and Yase, 1986).

Two hypotheses of an environmental cause for the ALS/PD/dementia complex of Guam are being investigated, both related to dietary factors and both claiming to be consistent with the declining incidence of the disease. One hypothesis favors the increased use of the seed of the false sago palm *cycas circinalis* as a foodstuff during the Japanese occupation during World War II, which would account for the increase in disease incidence following the war and a subsequent decline as the diet has become westernized (Spencer *et al.*, 1987). The other hypothesis (Garruto and Yase, 1986) is based on the unusually low concentrations of calcium and magnesium and relatively high concentrations of aluminum in the soil and water, especially in areas of high incidence in Guam. This hypothesis suggests a pathological accumulation of brain aluminum is responsible for the syndrome. A recent reassessment of the epidemiological patterns of the disease failed to show any association with mineral content of the water and soil, but reaffirmed an association with the use of cycad (Zhang *et al.*, 1990). Two potential neurotoxins – cycasin and B-N-methylamino-L-alanine (BMAA) – have been identified in the cycad seed and are being studied as the agent possibly responsible for this long-latency neurodegenerative disease (Spencer *et al.*, 1991).

Differences in geographic prevalence rates have been interpreted as supporting environmental factors in the etiology of idiopathic parkinsonism. Wherever investigated, idiopathic parkinsonism has been found in all ethnic groups (Schoenberg, 1987; Rajput *et al.*, 1984; Li *et al.*, 1985; Cosnett and Bill, 1988; Aquilonius and Hartvig, 1986). In general, prevalence rates are higher in industrialized western countries than in less developed countries (Tanner *et al.*, 1987; Schoenberg, 1987; Lux and Kurtzke, 1987). Door-to-door surveys in China (49/100 000) (Li *et al.*, 1985) and Nigeria (67/100 000) (Schoenberg *et al.*, 1988) support the thesis that the lower prevalence rate in these relatively non-industrialized countries is from an absence of those environmental factors associated with industrialization which predispose to the development of Parkinson's disease. A possible exception to this is a recent report of a door-to-door survey of the Parsi community in Bombay (Bharuca *et al.*, 1988) where the prevalence (328/100 000) is among the highest reported.

Another possible contradiction to the industrialization hypothesis is the increased risk of young-onset parkinsonism in North America in persons living in rural areas and drinking well water (Tanner and Langston, 1990). This may not be a contradiction, however, if herbicides and pesticides, which are used to a much greater extent in industrialized countries, are the offending agents. Some reports suggest an association of idiopathic parkinsonism with various occupational or residential exposures to pesticides, heavy metal or steel alloy industries, vegetable farming and wood pulp mills (Tanner, 1989). These studies vary in the rigor of their epidemiologic methods, and no consistent association with an environmental factor that can explain the worldwide distribution of the disease is apparent. Moreover, it has been argued that the stability of the incidence rates over 40 years in Rochester, Minnesota – where the prevalence rate is among the highest recorded – is against an environmental cause (Duvoisin, 1982; Eldridge *et al.*, 1986), since most industrial or agricultural chemicals were introduced relatively recently. However, we cannot discount the possibility of multiple environmental factors acting on individuals whose dopaminergic neurons are more susceptible to injury by virtue of aging or genetic factors.

19.   The interplay of genetic and environmental factors may play a role in the cause of idiopathic parkinsonism

It has not been possible to marshall convincing evidence that heredity or a specific environmental exposure are sufficient by themselves to cause idiopathic parkinsonism, but recent data have raised the possibility of a genetic susceptibility to exogenous or endogenous toxins (Johnson, 1991). One theory (the 'mitochondrial hypothesis') suggests that a maternally inherited defect in the mitochondrial genome results in inadequate detoxification of environmental toxins which, in turn, damage nigral neurons (Di Monte, 1991). Another suggested mechanism is a defect in the regulation of the oxidative metabolism of dopamine resulting in the excess generation or defective removal of free radicals ('free radical hypothesis') (Olanow, 1990). Both of these hypotheses take their cue from the observation that the mechanism of damage to the nigral neuron by MPTP is through the oxidation of MPTP to MPP+, which prevents the generation of ATP by inhibiting complex I in the mitochondria. The damage to the mitochondria and the dopaminergic neuron can be prevented by pretreatment with a MAO inhibitor to inhibit the oxidative deamination of MPTP to MPP+ (maxim 21). The mitochondrial hypothesis focuses on a mitochondrial defect that could be the result of exposure to a toxin with effects similar to MPP+ or a defect in the mitochondrial genome or a combination of both. The free radical hypothesis emphasizes the potential damage to lipid neuronal membranes from excess free radicals generated by the oxidative metabolism of dopamine. These two hypotheses are not mutually exclusive. Because the oxidative metabolism of dopamine produces potentially damaging free radicals and toxic metabolites, the substantia nigra is subjected to a high degree of oxidative stress. Any defect in the mitochondrial mechanisms regulating this process, whether genetic or produced by an environmental toxin, could upset the homeostasis of the system.

Three groups have reported abnormalities in mitochondrial function in patients with idiopathic parkinsonism (Schapira et al., 1990; Mizuno et al., 1989; Parker et al., 1989). A reduction of the activity of complex I has been demonstrated in postmortem specimens of striatum and substantia nigra and in the platelets of patients with idiopathic parkinsonism. The reason for this deficiency in complex I is unknown, but an abnormality in the mitochondrial or nuclear genome (both are involved in the coding of various subunits of complex I) could be postulated. As noted above (maxim

17), genetic studies have failed to provide support for either a Mendelian pattern of inheritance or maternal inheritance of a defect in mitochondrial DNA. However, a maternal pattern of inheritance might be difficult to detect if an environmental trigger was required to express the defect.

The evidence suggesting that oxidative stress may contribute to the pathogenesis of idiopathic parkinsonism is summarized in Table 19.1 (Olanow, 1990). Iron, which catalyzes oxidation reactions, is found in increased concentration in the substantia nigra of patients with idiopathic parkinsonism. Ferritin, the protein that binds and transports iron, is decreased in the brain of PD patients, implying that iron is present in a free form that would lead to an increase in oxidation reactions and free radical formation. Glutathione and glutathione peroxidase, which are responsible for detoxifying the hydrogen peroxide generated from dopamine metabolism, are reduced in the substantia nigra of patients with idiopathic parkinsonism. This development might reduce the capacity to prevent the formation of increased free radicals and lipid peroxidation. Evidence of increased lipid peroxidation in the substantia nigra of idiopathic parkinsonism patients has been reported. Finally, the possible protective effect of antioxidant agents provide additional support for the oxidative stress hypothesis (see maxim 38).

Decreased activity of an enzyme that detoxifies drugs by sulfate conjugation has also been reported in patients with idiopathic parkinsonism (Williams *et al.*, 1991), again raising the possibility that patients with idiopathic parkinsonism are more susceptible to environmental toxins.

Table 19.1 Evidence supporting oxidation reactions as a possible pathogenetic mechanism

Increased iron in the substantia nigra of patients with Parkinson's disease (PD)
Decreased ferritin in the brain of patients with PD
Decreased glutathione in the substantia nigra of patients with PD
Increased lipid peroxidation in the substantia nigra of patients with PD
Evidence that selegiline slows progression of parkinsonism
Decreased complex I in the substantia nigra and platelets of patients with PD

Modified from Olanow (1990)

20. *Always consider the possibility of drug-induced parkinsonism*

Because drug-induced parkinsonism is reversible with cessation of the offending drug, this cause of parkinsonism must always be considered (Weiner and Lang, 1989). Drugs that interfere with any step in dopaminergic neurotransmission can produce parkinsonism (Table 20.1). Drugs affecting presynaptic mechanisms by inhibition of synthesis of dopamine (alpha methyl paratyrosine), disruption of vesicular storage of dopamine (reserpine), or the production of false transmitters (alpha methyldopa) are now uncommon causes of parkinsonism. Drug-induced parkinsonism is most commonly caused by neuroleptics and other dopamine antagonists that block the striatal postsynaptic dopamine receptors.

Few physicians fail to recognize this potential of antipsychotic drugs, but dopamine antagonists used for gastrointestinal complaints may be overlooked. Metoclopramide in particular is becoming a more frequent and often overlooked cause of parkinsonism in the elderly. Trimethobenzamide, (Tigan) prochlorperazine, (Compazine), and chlorpromazine (Thorazine) used as an antiemetic are occasionally implicated. Antiemetics with central dopamine antagonist activity should not be used to treat the gastrointestinal side-effects of levodopa.

Drug combinations used for anxiety and depression may contain neuroleptics. The tricyclic dibenzoxazepine, amoxapine, is used as an antide-

Table 20.1   Drugs that produce parkinsonism

Antipsychotics (partial list of representative drugs)	A. phenothiazines
	1. trifluoperazine
	2. perphenazine
	3. fluphenazine
	B. Butyrophenones
	1. haloperidol
	2. droperidol
	C. Dibenzoxaphine
	1. loxapine
	D. Thiothanxene
	1. thiothixine
Antiemetics	A. Metoclopramide
	B. Proclorperazine
	C. Trimethobenzamide
Antihypertensives	A. Reserpine
	B. Alpha methyldopa
Antidepressants	A. Amoxapine
Calcium channel antagonists	A. Flunarizine
	B. Cinnarizine
Others	A. Well documented
	1. tetrabenazine
	2. alpha methylparatyrosine
	B. Rare or poorly documented
	1. lithium
	2. phenytoin
	3. captopril
	4. cytosine arabinoside

pressant, but a metabolite, loxapine, is an antipsychotic (Loxitane®) and produces all the extrapyramidal reactions of dopamine receptor antagonists including parkinsonism. Two calcium channel antagonists used in Europe, flunarizine and cinnarizine, have structural similarities to neuroleptics and cause parkinsonism.

One should always be alert to the possibility that a deterioration in treated or untreated parkinsonism may be due to the inadvertent addition of one of these drugs to the patient's medication regimen.

The only option for eliminating parkinsonism caused by drugs acting presynaptically is withdrawal of the drug. Withdrawal of dopamine antagonists is often not an option because the drug is necessary to control psychotic symptoms, in which case the lowest effective dose of an antipsychotic drug with low to medium potency should be used. Centrally acting anticholinergic drugs and amantadine ameliorate the parkinsonism caused by neuroleptics. Anticholinergics and amantadine can often be withdrawn after a few months as the nervous system adapts and nigrostriatal neurotransmission is restored in spite of the continued presence of the neuroleptic. Improvement in the parkinsonism may appear slowly after discontinuing dopamine antagonists – sometimes requiring months before the patient returns to baseline.

21.   *Neurotoxins can produce parkinsonism*

MPTP is the first neurotoxin to selectively damage the substantia nigra and produce signs and symptoms virtually indistinguishable from idiopathic parkinsonism. It also produces the clinical equivalent of the human condition in monkeys (Burns *et al.*, 1983; Forno *et al.*, 1986; Crossman *et al.*, 1987), providing an experimental model for study of the disease. Pathologically, it differs from the idiopathic disease by the pattern of cell loss in the substantia nigra and the absence of unequivocal Lewy bodies. It is a relatively simple compound related to other industrial and 'natural' chemicals (e.g. Paraquat, a herbicide, and pyridines, present in cigarette smoke), raising the possibility that exposure to an MPTP-like molecule in our environment may be critical for the development of idiopathic parkinsonism (maxim 18).

The selectivity of MPTP for the pigmented neurons of the substantia nigra is unique, but the basal ganglia are vulnerable to the neurotoxic effects of other agents, such as manganese and carbon disulfide, and to hypoxia and respiratory electron transport poisons such as carbon monoxide and cyanide (Table 15.1). The basal ganglia lesion is usually maximal in the globus pallidus and substantia nigra reticulata (Hawker and Lang, 1990). Although parkinsonian signs may predominate, other neurologic signs betray evidence of damage to other parts of the brain. For example, workers exposed to manganese in mining, smelting and steel industries experience behavioral changes and dystonia (Barbeau, 1984). Parkinsonian symptoms and signs have been reported in workers exposed to carbon disulfide in the rayon industry and to carbon disulfide-containing fumigants in grain storage facilities (Lewy, 1941; Peters *et al.*, 1982). The use of fumigants containing carbon disulfide has been discontinued and improved production practices and precautions have reduced exposure in the rayon industry. Carbon monoxide intoxication from an acute exposure more often produces manifestations of cortical damage (apraxia, agnosia, dementia) than basal ganglia involvement (parkinsonism) (Garland and Pearce, 1967). There is no convincing evidence that chronic exposure to subintoxicating levels of carbon monoxide produces parkinsonism.

Symmetric pallidal lesions and parkinsonism have also been seen in patients recovering from attempted suicide by drug overdose, during which there is a presumed hypoxic/ischemic injury from respiratory depression and hypotension (Hawker and Lang, 1990).

22.   *The parkinsonism plus syndromes account for 15% of all parkinsonism*

'Parkinsonism plus' syndromes refer to disorders in which the classical signs of parkinsonism are combined with other signs of neurological dysfunction, particularly autonomic, cerebellar, oculomotor or cortical.

These syndromes are estimated to compose 15% of the patients attending movement disorder clinics (Rajput *et al.*, 1984). Early in the course these cases may be impossible to distinguish from idiopathic parkinsonism. Parkinsonism plus syndromes may be suspected if there is (1) prominent akinesia and rigidity without tremor at onset, (2) rapid progression, or (3) development of neurologic signs indicating disease outside the basal ganglia. In many cases the first clue is a transient or poor response

Table 22.1   'Parkinsonism plus' syndromes

Progressive supranuclear palsy
Multiple system atrophy
1. Shy-Drager syndrome
2. Olivopontocerebellar degeneration
3. Striatonigral degeneration
Corticobasal degeneration
ALS/PD/dementia complex of Guam
Alzheimer's disease
Pick's disease
Diffuse Lewy body disease

to levodopa, which should alert one to look for the development of the other non-parkinsonian signs. Most of these cases turn out to have disorders in which the parkinsonism is the result of the degeneration of striatal and pallidal neurons in addition to nigral neurons. Dopaminergic therapy fails because the neurons in striatum that are the targets of the nigral dopaminergic output are no longer capable of responding. The prognosis for this group of patients is worse than for idiopathic parkinsonism.

It should be noted that patients with typical 'Lewy body disease' may sometimes have a rapidly progressive rigid bradykinetic syndrome that is unresponsive to levodopa.

23. Visual symptoms and impairment of eye movements suggest another disorder

A variety of eye signs may be noted in parkinsonism, but most of them are minor and cause no symptoms (Table 23.1). Visual complaints are uncommon, but if present usually relate to reading, probably because of impairment of visual tracking.

Prominent visual symptoms and impairment of eye movements, particularly downgaze, are most characteristic of progressive supranuclear palsy (PSP) (Steele et al., 1964; Maher and Lees, 1986) (Table 23.2). An inability to look down causes difficulty in walking over uneven ground or steps and curbs and in tying shoes. Eating may be impaired because the patient cannot look down to find the food on the plate.

Degeneration of supranuclear pathways in thalamus and midbrain responsible for initiation and control of eye movements accounts for the characteristic slowing and then paralysis of voluntary eye movements. Typically the patient first loses the ability to voluntarily direct the eyes downward, although down pursuit may be preserved. Subsequently all vertical movements are lost and horizontal movements are slowed. Finally the patient may be left with immobile eyes. Reflex ocular movements are preserved. In fact, the oculocephalic reflexes, which are normally suppressed in an awake person, are very easy to elicit, similar to what one

Table 23.1   Eye signs in parkinsonism

Decreased blink rate
Hypometric saccades
Impaired smooth pursuit
Reflex blepharosphasm (glabeller, Meyerson's sign)
Spontaneous blepharospasm
Oculogyric crises (postencephalitic parkinsonism)

would expect in a comatose patient with intact brainstem function. In addition to the defect in ocular motility, the patient has an impairment of orienting responses, with failure to turn the head or body toward the target or center of attention. Sometimes the diagnosis can be made upon entering the examining room when the patient responds to your greeting without turning their head or eyes to look at you.

Many patients complain of a decrease in visual acuity and difficulty reading, but visual acuity is normal when formally tested and lenses fail to improve the symptoms. This complaint may be due to pathology in the superior colliculus. Other ocular signs that may occur in PSP are listed in Table 23.2.

Bradykinesia and rigidity are the most common parkinsonian signs in PSP. A typical tremor is seldom if ever present. The rigidity in PSP has a different distribution from that typical of idiopathic parkinsonism. It affects the neck and axial musculature to produce an upright and even extended posture of the neck and shoulders and involves proximal limbs with relative sparing of distal muscles. An impairment of postural reflexes is usually prominent. Unlike idiopathic parkinsonism, many patients present with falling as an early symptom. Patients often inexplicably lose their balance, typically falling backwards with little effort to avert the fall, toppling over like a statue (see maxim 27). A pseudobulbar palsy frequently develops later in the course but is occasionally an early symptom or finding.

Most patients with PSP respond poorly or not at all to antiparkinsonian medications. However, an occasional patient derives a symptomatically useful improvement and medication trials should be offered. Levodopa or dopamine agonists may partially relieve parkinsonian symptoms. Patients who fail to respond to levodopa may still benefit from dopamine agonists (Jackson *et al.*, 1983). Anticholinergics and methysergide have been

Table 23.2   Eye signs in progressive supranuclear palsy (PSP)

Supranuclear ophthalmoplegia	+++
Early Impaired up and down gaze Hypometric horizontal saccades Slowed horizontal pursuit	
Late Ophthalmoplegia of vertical followed by horizontal gaze	
Reflex blepharospasm (glabellar, Meyerson's sign)	++
Spontaneous blepharospasm	++
Decreased blink rate	++
Easily elicited vestibulo-ocular reflex	++
Lid apraxia/involuntary levator inhibition	+
Internuclear opthalmoplegia	+

+++ Essential feature   ++ Common   + Less Common

reported to help pseudobulbar symptoms (Rafal and Grimm, 1981). Special prisms and ocular mirrors obtained from ophthalmologists or oculists can be helpful in looking down to read and eat. Reading stands can relieve the patient of looking down or wearing out their arms. The prognosis for PSP is much worse than idiopathic parkinsonism, survival averaging about eight years (Golbe *et al.*, 1988).

Late-onset hereditary or sporadic cerebellar ataxia (also referred to as olivopontocerebellar atrophy in some classifications) is usually not mistaken for parkinsonism, but occasionally parkinsonian hypomimea, bradykinesia and rigidity are present. If a patient has nystagmus and/or prominent slowing of pursuit and saccadic eye movements, look for limb and gait ataxia (see maxim 27).

24.   *Babinski signs in parkinsonism should alert the clinician to other entities*

Babinski signs are not part of the syndrome of idiopathic parkinsonism and if present should trigger a search for another disorder. One alternative might be the parkinsonism plus syndrome (e.g. multiple systems atrophy; see maxim 25), or a coincident disorder, such as spondylitic myelopathy. Fortunately for the patient, modern technology has made extensive invasive workups unnecessary. CT scan of the head may disclose an old stroke, the most common cause of a unilateral Babinski sign. MRI of the cervical spine can reveal a spondylitic myelopathy, the most common treatable cause of bilateral Babinski signs in this age group.

One must also be certain that a true Babinski sign is being elicited. A common mistake is to interpret a dystonic dorsiflexion of the great toe as a Babinski sign. This 'striatal toe' may be present in any disorder of the basal ganglia and can be discriminated from a Babinski sign by the fact that the extension of the toe is prolonged or tonic and occurs spontaneously, unrelated to any stimulus, although it may be present more frequently in certain positions or movements of the extremity. The response of the toe is normally flexor to plantar stimulation.

25.   *Early autonomic symptoms suggest multiple systems atrophy*

Although Lewy body degeneration of autonomic neurons is a regular feature of idiopathic parkinsonism, autonomic dysfunction generally becomes symptomatic years after the diagnosis of parkinsonism has been established. If orthostatic hypotension, impotence, or neurogenic bladder are early or prominent features, one should consider the diagnosis of multiple system atrophy. As the name implies, multiple neuronal systems in addition to the nigrostriatal system are involved in the degenerative process. This collection of disorders has been described with different names depending on which system is most affected, but because of considerable overlap in clinical and pathologic features it is currently customary to lump them together under the rubric 'multiple system atrophy' (MSA) (Quinn, 1989). They are best distinguished from each other by their presenting clinical signs (Table 25.1) and from idiopathic parkinsonism by the presence of cerebellar, motor neuron signs, neuropathy, or autonomic dysfunction and ultimately by the failure to respond to treatment with dopaminergic drugs. MRI will frequently show atrophy of the brainstem and cerebellum.

In contrast to the other subtypes of MSA which present with somatic neurological signs (parkinsonism, cerebellar, corticospinal signs) the Shy–Drager syndrome is notable for initial dysautonomia that may be present for up to three years before parkinsonian signs appear (Shy and Drager, 1960). Impotence in males, orthostatic hypotension, anhidrosis, and urinary frequency, nocturia, retention and overflow incontinence secondary to an atonic urinary bladder are the most common early symptoms. The significance of impotence in this age group may be difficult to evaluate and bladder symptoms are often confused with prostatism. Constipation is prominent; however, rectal incontinence can occur because of a lax anal sphincter. Orthostatic hypotension is common and disabling. Characteristically, the patient is asymptomatic while lying or sitting, but the blood pressure progressively falls as long as the patient remains erect, eventually leading to a faint.

The next stage is characterized by the appearance of the motor manifestations, including parkinsonism, cerebellar signs, corticospinal signs and

Table 25.1 Multiple system atrophies

| Common name | Clinical features | |
	Early	Late
Shy-Drager syndrome	Dysautonomia	Parkinsonism Cerebellar Motor neuron signs with amyotrophy and corticospinal signs Ocular palsies Dementia
Olivopontocerebellar atrophy	Cerebellar plus parkinsonism	Dysautonomia Corticospinal signs
Striatonigral degeneration	Parkinsonism	Dysautonomia Cerebellar signs

amyotrophy of distal muscles consistent with motor neuron involvement, slowing of ocular movements or frank ocular palsies, and stridor secondary to abductor vocal cord dysfunction. Other symptoms and signs of autonomic dysfunction (Table 25.2) may appear at any time in the course of the disorder. A respiratory disturbance that we have found characteristic is erratic, sighing inspirations. Other central respiratory disorders may ensue, including sleep apnea. Apneustic breathing has occurred in the terminal phase of the illness. Dementia may appear in the later stages, but is usually mild and may represent hypoxic/ischemic insults from the severe orthostatic hypotension.

The office diagnosis depends on the clinical examination demonstrating somatic neurological signs and the confirmation of orthostatic hypotension and a hypotonic neurogenic bladder. Supine and standing blood pressures are taken after waiting at least three minutes in each position. A significant drop is usually defined as >30 mmHg systolic or >20 mmHg mean arterial pressure. The lack of change of the heart rate with a change in body position and hypotension is characteristic of a loss in sympathetic tone and differentiates this disorder from orthostasis due to hypovolemia. A urodynamic evaluation should reveal an atonic neurogenic bladder and help to rule out an obstructive uropathy in males.

The tests of autonomic dysfunction which are required to differentiate MSA – before somatic neurological signs are apparent – from progressive autonomic failure (PAF, also known as idiopathic orthostatic hypotension) are sophisticated and require a special laboratory (Cohen *et al.*, 1987). The results depend on the site of the autonomic neuronal degeneration – i.e. whether it is preganglionic (MSA) or postganglionic (PAF). PAF, however, is rarely associated with parkinsonism.

Table 25.2 Autonomic symptoms and signs in PD and MSA

	PD	MSA
Orthostatic hypotension	++	+++
Urinary urgency and frequency	++	++
Urinary retention	+	+++
Impotence	+	+++
Constipation	++	+++
Rectal incontinence	0	+++
Loss of rectal sphincter tone	0	++
Hyperhidrosis	+	0
Anhidrosis	0	++
Impairment of temperature control	0	++
Iris atrophy	0	+
Dysphagia	+	++
Sighing respirations	0	++

+++ Common and/or disabling   ++ Relatively common, but seldom disabling   + Uncommon or mild   0 Absent or rare

In addition to autonomic, pyramidal and cerebellar dysfunction, other clues that raise suspicion in favor of MSA are early instability and falls, irregular jerky tremor, abnormal slowing of eye movements beyond that expected in idiopathic parkinsonism, severe dysarthria/dysphonia, deep limb pain unrelieved by levodopa, and a severe antecollis that interferes with feeding and swallowing (Table 25.3).

The response of the parkinsonian symptoms in MSA to dopaminergic drugs is quite variable, but is usually poor and unsatisfactory. A severe persistent intolerance to levodopa is common. Some patients experience a paradoxical worsening of tremor, bradykinesia, or rigidity in response to levodopa. Small doses may produce dyskinesia, worsening of the central respiratory disorder, or dysphonia. Anticholinergics have not been helpful. The disturbances in autonomic function, particularly orthostatic hypotension, produce the most disabling symptoms and the greatest therapeutic challenges in the early to middle stages of the disease (see maxim 83). Although the disease is often slowly progressive, the prognosis is generally much worse than idiopathic parkinsonism. Frequently these patients spend the last few years of their life wheelchair bound and can stay erect only long enough for short excursions between rooms in their house. Because of the progressive loss of central regulation of cardiorespiratory function, sudden death is not unusual. Tracheostomy has been helpful in some cases of vocal cord paralysis and sleep apnea.

Table 25.3 Other clinical features of MSA

Early postural instability and falls
Rapid progression
Irregular jerky tremor
Myoclonus
Abnormal eye movements
Severe dysarthria and dysphonia
Pain unrelieved by levodopa
Disproportionate antecollis
Poor or absent response to levodopa
Severe levodopa intolerance

Source: After Quinn (1989)

26. *Prominent apraxia or rigidity suggests corticobasal degeneration*

First described as 'corticodentatonigral degeneration with neuronal achromasia' (Rebeiz *et al.*, 1968) and more recently as corticobasal ganglionic or simply corticobasal degeneration (Gibb *et al.*, 1989; Riley *et al.*, 1990), this uncommon disorder is differentiated from idiopathic parkinsonism and

PSP by the presence of symptoms and signs of frontal and parietal cortical dysfunction in addition to the basal ganglia signs. The most characteristic combination is apraxia and rigidity starting in one limb which spreads to the other ipsilateral limb and then the contralateral limbs over a period of a few years. For unknown reasons, it usually begins in the nondominant arm. Initially the apraxia may be overlooked because the clumsiness of the hand is assumed to be due to the rigidity and bradykinesia. Eventually the apraxia becomes more apparent, rendering the hand useless. The limb may also have the curious habit of assuming bizarre postures or interfere with actions of the good hand as if it had a mind of its own, the 'alien hand syndrome'. Apraxia of a leg may present as a gait disorder resulting from a disturbance of proper placing and sequencing of stepping. Falling may result from a failure to put the foot down after lifting it to step. Cortical sensory loss, constructional apraxia, dysarthria and frontal lobe release signs are common.

Basal ganglia involvement is manifested by marked rigidity, brady-kinesia, and masked facies. A tremor is often present, but is not a typical resting tremor. The tremor is a fine, rapid, irregular tremor that is increased by active or passive movement of the limb. It may be myoclonic rather than a true tremor and may be elicited by a tap of the fingers. EEG back averaging in one case was consistent with a cortical reflex myoclonus (Riley et al., 1990). Occasionally chorea or dystonia are present.

A supranuclear gaze disturbance may develop, but does not preferentially affect downgaze nor is it as prominent as in PSP. Dementia may occur later in the course, but the prominent motor signs differentiate corticobasal degeneration from Alzheimer's disease. MRI and CT scans sometimes show asymmetric focal atrophy of parietal cortex contralateral to the limb first and most severely affected (Riley et al., 1990).

The characteristic pathology of autopsied cases is neuronal loss and gliosis of paracentral frontal and parietal cortex and substantia nigra. Characteristic pale, swollen neurons (neuronal achromasia) are found in cortex (Rebeiz et al., 1968). Lightly basophilic cytoplasmic inclusions are sometimes seen in surviving neurons (Gibb et al., 1989). Other features of Pick's disease, Alzheimer's disease or idiopathic parkinsonism are not present.

Treatment with levodopa dopamine agonists or anticholinergics is of no benefit. Clonazepam can suppress the tremor or myoclonus, but produces no functional improvement. The course is relentless until the patient is akinetic and anarthric in 5–8 years.

27.   *Gait disturbance and falling are not prominent early symptoms of idiopathic parkinsonism*

Although marked abnormalities of gait and loss of postural reflexes with falling may become the serious disabilities late in the course of idiopathic parkinsonism, they are not prominent at the onset of symptoms. In the early stages of idiopathic parkinsonism, the gait and postural reflexes are virtually normal. There may be a slight lag or dragging of one foot. More commonly the first abnormalities are a decrease in arm swing and mild flexion posturing of one arm. As the disease advances to the later stages the trunk adopts a flexed posture and the stride becomes shortened with the feet sliding along the floor. There is frequent freezing with difficulty initiating gait as if the foot were stuck to the floor (start hesitation). The stride becomes short, quick steps on the toes (festination) (Table 27.1), especially as the patient approaches a doorway or step. Instead of turning with a smart pivot with the head leading the way, the entire body rotates as a rigid unit directly over the feet and requires a few steps to accomplish the turn as if rotating on a pedestal (en bloc turn). The gait improves if the patient has a long straight course to walk and deteriorates if he has to turn or maneuver in tight quarters, such as an examining room. If the patient's attention is distracted while he is walking, he may freeze or lose his balance and fall.

While start hesitation, freezing and en bloc turns are commonly seen in idiopathic parkinsonism, these abnormalities are by no means specific to this disorder. The mult-infarct state, for example, or normal pressure hydrocephalus (NPH) may also cause a variety of abnormalities of gait and often cause diagnostic confusion. There are clues that differentiate these disorders from idiopathic parkinsonism. In contrast to idiopathic parkinsonism, the base is often widened in a multi-infarct gait disorder. The less severely affected patient with multi-infarct gait disorder who can still walk unaided assumes an upright posture, and arm swing is retained with the

Table 27.1 Syndromes with prominent gait disturbance

Disease	Base	Freezing	Festina-tion	Falling	Dys-metria
Late parkinsonism	Normal	+++	+++	+	0
PSP	Normal	+	0	+++	0
MSA	Normal or wide	+	+	++	++
Lacunar state	Normal or wide	+++	0	++	0
Hydrocephalus	Normal or wide	++	+	++	+
Frontal lesion	Normal or wide	++	+	++	+

+++ invariably present   ++ common   + sometimes present   0 absent arms extended at the elbows (Thompson and Marsden, 1987). There is start hesitation and shuffling, but no festination. Turning is particularly laborious with the patient sometimes using one foot as a pivot around which he pushes himself with the other. Also unlike the parkinsonian, one foot may always lead the other and alternate stepping is impossible. In the early stages of vascular parkinsonism the postural reflexes are preserved. More advanced cases stand on stiffly extended legs with feet firmly 'glued' to the floor. When an attempt is made to step forward the multi-infarct patient bends forward reaching for support and develops increasing sway of the trunk before losing his balance. Later these patients cannot stand unaided. They lose all sense of an upright posture; the patient defeats all attempts by the examiner to push and encourage him to an erect posture by remaining flexed at the hips and knees and stepping forward while leaning backwards fully supported by the examiner. The gait disorder associated with the multi-infarct state has been referred to by many different names: 'marché à petit pas', magnetic gait, frontal lobe apraxia, 'slipped clutch', or 'lower half parkinsonism' (Thompson and Marsden, 1987; Fitz-Gerald and Jankovic, 1989).

While disturbance of gait is the principal symptom of NPH, the gait disturbance can vary considerably in severity and type, from a mild unsteadiness suggesting a cerebellar ataxia, to a marked shuffling, freezing and falling that resembles severe parkinsonism (Fisher, 1982). In comparison with patients with idiopathic parkinsonism, patients with NPH more often complain of a disabling weakness and tiredness of the legs with standing or walking. Although the gait disorder is the primary symptom in NPH, urinary urgency and incontinence, and cognitive dysfunction appear later to complete the typical clinical triad of this disorder.

Other clues that differentiate gait disorders due to idiopathic parkinsonism from those caused by multiple strokes or NPH are the paucity of other unequivocal signs of parkinsonism. Rest tremor, bradykinesia, and true rigidity are absent, especially in the upper extremities. The gait disorder appears to be out of proportion to any other motor signs, and incongruously arm swing is retained or even exaggerated. The presence of corticospinal signs (spasticity, hyperreflexia, Babinski signs) especially in the legs are helpful clues. The presence of dementia and/or incontinence are other indicators in favor of another diagnosis (see maxim 28). However, rarely, both hydrocephalus (Jankovic et al., 1986) and multiple lacunes (Murrow et al., 1990) can produce a parkinsonian syndrome that is responsive to levodopa and indistinguishable from idiopathic parkinsonism.

CT and MR scans are often helpful in identifying the lacunar state, NPH or frontal lesions. NPH may be suspected when the CT scan shows ventriculomegaly (including the temporal horns of the lateral ventricles), absence of cortical atrophy, and periventricular hypointensity at the angles of the frontal horns. However, no CT or MRI scan is diagnostic for NPH, as judged by the gold standard of the response to CSF shunting. Isotope cisternograms or transient CSF drainage may help identify candidates more likely to respond to shunting. In the multi-infarct state the MRI shows patchy white matter lesions with lacunar infarcts in the basal ganglia and brainstem.

Parkinsonism with an early and prominent disturbance in standing and walking balance is characteristic of progressive supranuclear palsy (maxim 23). Falling for no apparent reason is an early symptom of PSP and may appear before the supranuclear gaze disturbance. The falling in this syndrome may also occur in the relative absence of the other disturbances of gait. The PSP patient may walk quite upright with a normal stride, stance and arm swing. The gait problem appears on turning, in which the patient does not appear to appreciate the center of gravity or even to recognize that he is falling; he pitches to the side or backwards, often not making any effort to recover or break the fall. Even while standing quietly the patient may drift to the side or backwards and then fall. This marked disturbance in postural reflexes can be readily demonstrated by pulling the patient forwards or backwards; the patient with PSP cannot recover and will invariably fall if not caught.

A staggering wide-based ataxic gait suggests a cerebellar degeneration. Although ataxia as an isolated finding offers little confusion with parkinsonism, cerebellar ataxia may be combined with parkinsonism in some of the multiple system atrophies, in particular olivopontocerebellar atrophy or the Shy–Drager syndrome. In addition to the ataxic gait and parkinsonian features one should see other evidence of cerebellar dysfunction such as nystagmus, cerebellar dysarthria and limb ataxia. The MRI scan frequently shows cerebellar and pontine atrophy.

28.   *Dementia is not an early symptom of idiopathic parkinsonism*

The prevalence of dementia in idiopathic parkinsonism is greater than the general population, but dementia is not an invariable part of the disease and is rarely an early symptom. If dementia occurs early in the course of the parkinsonian syndrome another cause is often responsible, in particular Alzheimer's disease (AD) or a multi-infarct dementia. In AD the parkinsonian features generally appear in the later stages of the disease and consist of bradykinesia and rigidity. Differentiating rigidity from the *gegenhalten* phenomenon (paratonia) is difficult and may account for reports of a high prevalence of parkinsonism in AD. Rest tremor, which is more specific for idiopathic parkinsonism, occurs in only about 5–10% of patients with AD (Gibb, 1989a). This clinical experience is in agreement with the pathological findings; cell loss, plaques and tangles in the substantia nigra are common but mild in AD. On the other hand, the prevalence of Lewy bodies in the substantia nigra is the same in AD as the general population. Antiparkinsonian medications rarely help these patients, and commonly increase confusion and behavioral abnormalities.

The multi-infarct or lacunar state with dementia is more difficult to distinguish from idiopathic parkinsonism because the motor signs may also precede the dementia. Lacunar state should be suspected when a gait disorder is the most prominent motor disability in persons at risk for cerebrovascular disease. Bilateral corticospinal signs are usually present. A history of stroke-like episodes, a pseudobulbar emotional lability, and incontinence are helpful in distinguishing multi-infarct state from idiopathic parkinsonism; these signs are not always present, however.

A combination of dementia (apathy and abulia), gait disorder, and parkinsonism also may be seen in frontal lobe tumors. Other parkinsonian syndromes with dementia – such as normal pressure hydrocephalus or parkinsonism plus syndromes – are listed in Table 28.1. Like idiopathic parkinsonism, the dementia in these conditions is generally mild and appears later in the course of the disorder after the motor signs are well established.

Table 28.1   Parkinsonism and dementia

Dementia > motor signs	Motor signs > dementia	Variable onset and severity of dementia in relation to motor signs
Alzheimer's disease	Idiopathic parkinsonism	Multi-infarct state
Pick's disease	Progressive supranuclear palsy	Huntington's disease
Frontal lobe tumor	Striatonigral degeneration	Cortical Lewy body
Pugilist's	Shy–Drager Syndrome	disease
encephalopathy	Corticobasal degeneration	
	Normal-pressure hydrocephalus	
	Parkinsonism–dementia	
	complex of Guam	
	Creutzfeldt–Jakob disease	
	Wilson's disease	
	Hallervorden Spatz disease	

29.   Vascular disease may produce parkinsonian features but seldom the complete syndrome of Parkinson's disease

Vascular disease as a cause of the syndrome of idiopathic parkinsonism has been debated since Critchley described atherosclerotic parkinsonism (Critchley, 1929). Critchley defined parkinsonism as nonpyramidal rigidity, weakness and slowness often accompanied by short stepped gait, pseudo-bulbar palsy, dementia, urinary incontinence and occasionally associated with cerebellar signs. Critchley recognized that most cases of atherosclerotic parkinsonism would not be confused with idiopathic parkinsonism.

Diagnostically, a history suggesting little strokes or stepwise progression of the gait disorder is helpful but often not present. The most helpful clinical features that distinguish vascular parkinsonism from idiopathic parkinsonism are the presence of corticospinal signs, pseudobulbar palsy, dementia, incontinence and other focal cortical signs. However, early presentation may be of a gait disorder and relative lack of parkinsonian signs, particularly tremor, in the upper body (FitzGerald and Jankovic, 1989). A lack of response to levodopa is also typical of vascular parkinsonism. Parkinsonism that spontaneously improves has been attributed to basal ganglia infarcts (Tolosa and Santamaria, 1984). The diagnosis rests on the demonstration of vascular lesions on CT or MR imaging of vascular parkinsonism.

An exception to the clinical rule dictums above was recently reported. A man with typical features of idiopathic parkinsonism including tremor and a good response to levodopa was found at autopsy to have a lacunar state without Lewy body degeneration of nigral neurons (Murrow *et al.*, 1990). It was hypothesized that the vascular disease had affected nigrostriatal projections without injuring the cell bodies.

It has been suggested that a significant proportion of patients with progressive supranuclear palsy have a multi-infarct state (Dubinsky and Jankovic, 1987). These authors found that 60% of 60 patients had hypertension and 32% had clinical or radiographic evidence of cerebrovascular disease. At autopsy, however, most patients with the clinical diagnosis of PSP have degenerative disorders.

30.   *A variety of other lesions of the basal ganglia may produce parkinsonism*

A variety of destructive lesions of the basal ganglia are uncommon causes of parkinsonism (Gibb, 1989b) (see Table 15.1). Parkinsonism and dystonia are regular features of Wilson's disease, a recessively inherited disorder of copper metabolism. If left untreated, virtually complete destruction of the putamen and globus pallidus may be a consequence. Another rare recessive disorder with features of dystonia and parkinsonism is Hallervorden–Spatz disease, which is associated with an excess accumulation of iron in basal ganglia. Parkinsonism is an uncommon feature of the adolescent and adult-onset cases of Leigh's disease, a rare mitochondrial disease that most commonly presents in infancy and childhood. Calcification of the basal ganglia and parkinsonism may be seen both in hypoparathyroidism and in a rare familial disorder (Fahr's disease). A rare association of basal ganglia calcification and a gait disorder resembling parkinsonism has been described in two patients with hyperparathyroidism (Margolin *et al.*, 1980) (Fig. 34.1). Lesser degrees of calcification of the basal ganglia are often an incidental finding and are generally unaccompanied by parkinsonian or other basal ganglia signs. Survivors of central pontine myelinolysis may show parkinsonism as a result of the extension of the lesion into the basal ganglia (Tinker *et al.*, 1990).

Even though head trauma is common, well documented reports of acute head trauma as a cause of parkinsonism are difficult to find (Factor *et al.*, 1988). On the other hand, bradykinesia and masked facies are often present in pugilistic or boxer's encephalopathy ('dementia pugilistica', 'punch drunk syndrome') and occasionally a typical resting tremor is seen (Critchley, 1957; Mawdsley and Ferguson, 1963).

After Von Economo's encephalitis disappeared, encephalitis has become a rare cause of parkinsonism. Occasional reports of parkinsonism in AIDS encephalopathy are now appearing (Nath *et al.*, 1987) and will probably become more frequent as the epidemic widens. Primary CNS lymphoma in the striatum is a rare cause, and other tumors are even more uncommon as a cause of idiopathic parkinsonism.

Among the miscellaneous causes of parkinsonism, an unusual syndrome of dystonia with parkinsonian features should be mentioned (Nygaard *et al.*, 1991). It characteristically begins in childhood and is usually familial,

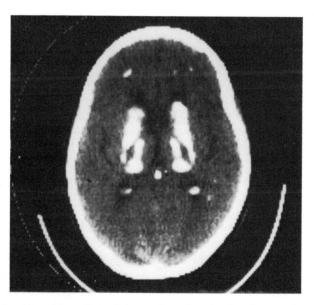

Fig. 34.1 Asymptomatic calcium deposits in basal ganglia are not uncommon in CT scans as an incidental finding. Rarely, dense calcification is associated with parkinsonism

although sporadic cases and onset in early adulthood have been reported. The hallmark of this particular disorder is a characteristic diurnal variation in the dystonic symptoms, which are responsive to low doses of levodopa (¼ – ½ tablet Sinemet 10/100 or 25/100 two to three times per day) hence the name dopa-responsive dystonia. Parkinsonism appearing in childhood is also seen in the rigid form of childhood-onset Huntington's disease.

31.   *The neurological workup is dictated by atypical historical features or neurological signs*

The diagnosis of idiopathic parkinsonism rests on the clinical history and exam alone; laboratory tests and imaging studies are directed at the exclusion of other causes of the syndrome. Like idiopathic parkinsonism, most other causes are diagnosed or suspected on the basis of a history and the physical examination. While MRI has not proven to be reliable for making the diagnosis of idiopathic parkinsonism, it has proven to be the single most useful test in looking for other etiologies. Imaging is indicated when there is a suspicion of a multi-infarct state, NPH, tumor or destructive metabolic or toxic lesion, such as Wilson's disease or CO poisoning. Brainstem and cerebellar atrophy may be evident on MR or CT scans in multiple system atrophy, and iron content of striatum (evidenced by a hypointense T2 weighted signal on high-field MRI) may be increased (Drayer *et al.*, 1986). In corticobasal degeneration the MRI may show cortical atrophy in the region of the Rolandic fissure contralateral to the first and most severely affected limb. A study of PSP has shown that a third of patients had MRI evidence of a multi-infarct state (Dubinsky and Jankovic, 1987), but this observation is not helpful diagnostically. Atrophy of the midbrain or enlargement of the aqueduct can be seen by MRI in some cases of PSP. Although caudate atrophy on CT may be seen in the rigid form of Huntington's disease, this finding is not always present. Unilateral Babinski signs should prompt a CT scan of the head, and bilateral Babinski signs an MRI of the cervical canal.

Chemistry tests are most commonly used to seek treatable causes of dementia with parkinsonism, especially hypothyroidism. If a CT scan shows calcification of the basal ganglia, the possibility of hyper- and hypoparathyroidism should be investigated with blood calcium, phosphorus and parathormone. Ceruloplasmin, urine and blood copper will screen for Wilson's disease. A Kayser–Fleischer ring is almost invariably present if neurologic signs are elicited, but it may require a slit-lamp exam by an ophthalmologist to see it.

References

Alexander GE, Crutcher MD. Functional architecture of basal ganglia circuits: neural substrates of parallel processing. *TINS* 1990; **13**: 266–71.

Aquilonius SM, Hartvig P. A Swedish county with unexpectedly high utilization of anti-parkinsonian drugs. *Acta Neurol Scand* 1986; **74**: 379–81.

Ballard PA, Tetrud TW, Langston JW. Permanent human parkinsonism due to 1-methyl-4-phenyl-1,2,3,6-tetrahydropyridine (MPTP): seven cases. *Neurology* 1985; **35**: 949–56.

Barbeau A. Manganese and extrapyramidal disorders. *Neurotoxicology* 1984; **5**: 13–36

Barbeau A, Roy M, Langston JW. Neurological consequence of industrial exposure to 1-methyl-4-phenyl-1,2,3,6-tetrahydropyridine. *Lancet* 1985; **1**: 747–7.

Bernheimer H, Birkmayer W, Hornykiewicz O, Jellinger K, Seitelberger F. Brain dopamine and the syndromes of Parkinson and Huntington–clinical, morphological and neurochemical correlations. *J Neurol Sci* 1973; **20**: 415–25.

Bharuca NE, Bharuca EP, Bharuca AE, Bhise AV, Schoenberg BS. Prevalence of Parkinson's disease in the Parsi community in Bombay, India. *Arch Neurol* 1988; **45**: 1321–4.

Burns RS, Chiueh CC, Markey SP, Ebert MH, Jacobowitz DM, Kopin IJ. A primate model of parkinsonism: selective destruction of dopaminergic neurons in the pars compacta of the substantia nigra by n-methyl-4-phenyl-1,2,3,6-tetrahydropyridine. *Proc Natl Acad Sci* 1983; **80**: 4546–50.

Burns RS, LeWitt PA, Ebert MH, Pakkenberg H, Kopin IJ. The clinical syndrome of striatal dopamine deficiency. Parkinsonism induced by 1-methyl-4-phenyl-1,2,3,6-tetrahydropyridine. *N Engl J Med* 1985; **312**: 1418–21.

Calne DB, Langston JW, Martin WRW, Stoessl AJ, Ruth TJ, Adam MJ, Pate BD and Schulzer M. Positron emission tomography after MPTP: observations relating to the cause of Parkinson's disease. *Nature* 1985; **317**: 246–48.

Calne DB. Is 'Parkinson's disease' one disease? *J Neurol Neurosurg Psychiat* 1989; (special suppl) 18–21.

Calne S, Schoenberg B, Martin WRW, Uitti RJ, Spencer P, Calne DB. Familial Parkinson's disease: possible role of environmental factors. *Can J Neurol Sci* 1987; **14**: 303–5.

Cohen J, Low P, Fealey R, Sheps S, Jiang N–S. Somatic and automatic function in progressive autonomic failure and multiple system atrophy. *Ann Neurol* 1987; **22**: 692–9.

Cosnett JE, Bill PLA. Parkinson's disease in blacks: observations on epidemiology in Natal. *S Afr Med J* 1988; **73**: 281–3.

Critchley M. Arteriosclerotic parkinsonism. *Brain* 1929; **52**: 23–83.

Critchley M. Medical aspects of boxing, particularly from a neurological standpoint. *Br Med J* 1957; **1**: 357–62.

Crossman AR, Clarke CE, Boyce S, Robertson RG, Sambrook MA. MPTP-induced Parkinsonism in the monkey: neurochemical pathology, complications of treatment and pathophysiological mechanisms. *Can J Neurol Sci* 1987; **14**: 428–35.

Davis GC, Williams AC, Markey SP. Chronic parkinsonism secondary to intravenous injection of meperidine analogues. *Psychiat Res* 1979; **1**: 249–54.

DeLong MR. Primate models of movement disorders of basal ganglia origin. *TINS* 1990; **13**: 281–54.

Di Monte D A. Mitochondrial DNA and Parkinson's disease. *Neurology* 1991; **41** (suppl 2): 38–42.

Drayer BP, Olanow W, Burger P, Johnson GA, Herfkens R, Riederer S. Parkinson plus syndrome: diagnosis using high-field MR imaging of brain iron. *Radiology* 1986; **159**: 493–8.

Dubinsky RM, Jankovic J. Progressive supranuclear palsy and a multi-infarct state. *Neurology* 1987; **37**: 570–6.

Duvoisin RC. On the cause of Parkinson's disease. In: Marsden CD and Fahns (eds), *Movement Disorders*. London: Butterworth Scientific 1982.

Eldridge R, Rocca WA, Ince S E. Parkinson's disease: evidence against toxic etiology and for an alternative theory. In: Markey S P, Castagnoli N, Trevor AJ, Kopin IJ (eds), *MPTP: A Neurotoxin Producing a Parkinsonian Syndrome*. New York: Academic Press, 1986: 355–67.

Factor S, Sanchez-Ramos J, Weiner W. Trauma as an etiology of parkinsonism: a historical review of the concept. *Movement Dis* 1988; **3** (1): 30.

Fisher CM. Hydrocephalus as a cause of disturbances of gait in the elderly. *Neurology* 1982; **32**: 1358–63.

FitzGerald PM, Jankovic J. Lower body parkinsonism: evidence for vascular etiology. *Movement Dis* 1989; **4**: 249–60.

Forno LS, Langston JW, DeLanney LE, Irwin I, Ricaurte GA. Locus ceruleus lesions and eosinophilic inclusions in MPTP-treated monkeys. *Ann Neurol* 1986; **20**: 449–55.

Garland H, Pearce J. Neurological complications of carbon monoxide poisoning. *Quart J Med* 1967; **36**: 445–55.

Garruto RM, Yase Y. Neurodegenerative disorders of the western Pacific: the search for mechanisms of pathogenesis. *TINS* 1986; Aug: 368–74.

Gibb WRG. Neuropathology in movement disorders. *J Neurol Neurosurg Psychiat* 1989a; **52** (special suppl): 55–67.

Gibb WRG. Dementia and Parkinson's disease. *Br J Psychiat* 1986; **154**: 596–614.

Gibb WRG, Lees AJ. The relevance of the Lewy body to the pathogenesis of idiopathic Parkinson's disease. *J Neurol Neurosurg Psychiat* 1988; **51**: 745–52.

Gibb WRG, Luthert PJ, Marsden CD. Corticobasal degeneration. *Brain* 1989; **112**: 1171–92.

Golbe LI. The genetics of Parkinson's disease: a reconsideration. *Neurology* 1990; **40** (suppl 3): 7–14.

Golbe LI, Davis PH, Schoenberg BS, Duvoisin RC. Prevalence and natural history of progressive supranuclear palsy. *Neurology* 1988; **38**: 1031–4.

Halliday GM, Li YW, Blumbergs PC, Joh TH, Cotton GH, Howe PRC, Blessing WW, Geffen, LB. Neuropathology of immunohistochemically identified brainstem neurons in Parkinson's disease. *Ann Neurol* 1990; **27**: 373–85.

Hawker K, Lang AE. Hypoxic–ischemic damage of the basal ganglia: case reports and a review of the literature. *Movement Dis* 1990; **5**: 219–24.

Hirano A. Electron microscopy in neuropathology. In: Zimmerman H (ed), *Progress in Neuropathology*. New York: Grune & Stratton, 1970: 1–61.

Jackson JA, Jankovic J, Ford J. Progressive supranuclear palsy: clinical features and response to treatment in 16 patients. *Ann Neurol* 1983; **13**: 273–8.

Jankovic JA, Newmark M, Peter P. Parkinsonism and acquired hydrocephalus. *Movement Dis* 1986; **1**: 59–64.

Jellinger K. The pathology of parkinsonism. In: Marsden CD, Fahn S (eds), *Movement Disorders 2*. London: Butterworths, 1987: 124–65.

Johnson WG. Genetic susceptibility to Parkinson's disease. *Neurology* 1991; **41** (suppl 2): 82–7.

Johnson WG, Hodge SE, Duvoisin R. Twin studies and the genetics of Parkinson's disease – a reappraisal. *Movement Dis* 1990; **5**: 187–94.

Langston JW, Ballard P. Parkinson's disease in a chemist working with 1-methyl-4-phenyl-1, 2, 3, 6-tetrahydropyridine. *N Engl J Med* 1983a; **309**: 747.

Langston JW, Ballard P., Tetrud JW, and Irwin I. Chronic parkinsonism in humans due to a product of meperidine-analog synthesis. *Science* 1983b; **219**: 979–80.

Lewy FH. Neurological, medical and biochemical signs and symptoms indicating chronic industrial carbon disulfide absorption. *Ann Internal Med* 1941; **15**: 869–83.

Li S, Schoenberg BS, Wang C, Cheng X, Rui D, Bolis L, Schoenberg DG. A prevalence survey of Parkinson's disease and other movement disorders in the People's Republic of China. *Arch Neurol* 1985; **42**: 655–7.

Lux WE, Kurtzke JF. Is Parkinson's disease acquired? Evidence from a geographic comparison with multiple sclerosis. *Neurology* 1987; **37**: 467–71.

Maher ER, Lees AJ. The clinical features and natural history of Steele-Richardson-Olszewski syndrome (progressive supranuclear palsy). *Neurology* 1986; **36**: 1005–8.

Margolin D, Hammerstad JP, Orwall E, McClung M, Calhoun D. Intracranial calcification in hyperparathyroidism: association with gait apraxia and parkinsonism. *Neurology* 1980; **30**: 1005–7.

Marsden CD. Parkinson's disease in twins. *J Neurol Neurosurg Psychiat* 1987; **50**: 105–6.

Marttila RJ, Kaprio J, Koskenvuo M, Rinne UK. Parkinson's disease in a nationwide twin cohort. *Neurology* 1988; **38**: 1217–19.

Mawdsley C, Ferguson FR. Neurological disease in boxers. *Lancet* 1963; **ii**: 795–801.

Mizuno Y, Ohta S, Tanaka M, Takamiya S, Suzuki K, Sato T, Oya H, Ozawa T, Kagawa Y. Deficiencies in complex I subunits of the respiratory chain in Parkinson's disease. *Biochem Biophys Res Commun* 1989; **163**: 1450–5.

Murrow RW, Schweiger GD, Kepes JJ, Koller WC. Parkinsonism due to a basal ganglia lacunar state: clinicopathologic correlation. *Neurology* 1990; **40**: 897–900.

Nath A, Jankovic J, Pettigrew LC. Movement disorders and AIDS. *Neurology* 1987; **37**: 37–41.

Nygaard TG, Marsden CD, Fahn S. Dopa-responsive dystonia: long-term treatment response and prognosis. *Neurology* 1991; **41**: 174–81.

Olanow CW. Oxidation reactions in Parkinson's disease. *Neurology* 1990; **40** (suppl 3): 32–7.

Parker WD, Boyson SJ, Park JK. Abnormalities of the electron transport chain in idiopathic Parkinson's disease. *Ann Neurol* 1989; **26**: 719–23.

Peters HA, Levine RL, Matthews CG, Sauter SL, Rankin JH. Carbon disulfide-induced neuropsychiatric changes in grain storage workers. *Am J Ind Med* 1982; **3**: 373–91.

Quinn N. Multiple system atrophy – the nature of the beast. *J Neurol Neurosurg Psychiat* 1989; **52** (special suppl): 78–89.

Rafal RD, Grimm RJ. Progressive supranuclear palsy: functional analysis of the response to methysergide and antiparkinsonian agents. *Neurology* 1981; **31**: 1507–18.

Rajput AH, Offord KP, Beard CM, Kurland LT. Epidemiology of parkinsonism: incidence, classification and mortality. *Ann Neurol* 1984; **16**: 278–82.

Rebeiz JJ, Kolodny EH, Richardson EP. Corticodentatonigral degeneration with neuronal achromasia. *Arch Neurol* 1968; **18**: 20–33.

Riley DE, Lang AE, Lewis A, Resch L, Ashby P, Hornykiewicz D, Black S. Cortical-basal ganglionic degeneration. *Neurology* 1990; **40**: 1203–12.

Robinson TE, Whishaw IQ. Normalization of extracellular dopamine in striatum following recovery from a partial unilateral 6-OHDOPA lesion of the substantia nigra: a microdialysis study in freely moving rats. *Brain Res* 1988; **450**: 209–24.

Sacks O. *Awakenings*. New York: HarperCollins, 1990.

Schapira AHV, Cooper JM, Dexter D, Clark JB, Jenner P, Marsden CD. Mitochondrial Complex I deficiency in Parkinson's disease. *J Neurochem* 1990; **54**: 823–7.

Schoenberg BS. Environmental risk factors for Parkinson's disease: the epidemiologic evidence. *Can J Neurol Sci* 1987; **14** (suppl): 407–13.

Schoenberg BS, Osuntokun BO, Adeuja AOG. Comparison of the prevalence of

Parkinson's disease in black populations in the rural US and in rural Nigeria: door-to-door community studies. *Neurology* 1988; **38**: 645–6.

Shy GM, Drager GA. A neurological syndrome associated with orthostatic hypotension. *Arch Neurol* 1960; **2**: 511–27.

Spencer PS. Guam ALS/parkinsonism-dementia: a long-latency neurotoxic disorder caused by slow toxin(s) in food? *Can J Neurol Sci* 1987; **14** (suppl): 347–57.

Spencer PS, Kisby GE, Ludolph AC. Slow toxins, biologic markers, and long-latency neurodegenerative disease in the western Pacific region. *Neurology* 1991; **41** (suppl 2): 62–6.

Spencer PS, Nunn PB, Hugon J, Ludolph AC, Ross SM, Roy DN, Robertson RC. Guam amyotrophic lateral sclerosis-parkinsonism-dementia linked to a plant excitant neurotoxin. *Science* 1987; **237**: 517–22.

Steele JC, Richardson JC, Olszewski J. Progressive supranuclear palsy: a heterogeneous degeneration involving brainstem, basal ganglia and cerebellum with vertical gaze and pseudobulbar palsy, nuchal dystonia and dementia. *Arch Neurol* 1964; **10**: 333–59.

Tanner CM. The role of environmental toxins in the etiology of Parkinson's disease. *Trends Neurosci* 1989; **12**: 49–52.

Tanner CM, Chen B, Wang WZ, Peng ML, Liuz L, Liang XL, Kao LC, Gilley DW, Schoenberg BS. Environmental factors in the etiology of Parkinson's disease. *Can J Neurol Sci* 1987; **14** (suppl): 419–23.

Tanner CM, Langston JW. Do environmental toxins cause Parkinson's disease? A critical review. *Neurology* 1990; **40** (suppl 3): 17–30.

Thompson PD, Marsden CD. Gait disorder of subcortical arteriosclerotic encephalopathy: Binswanger's disease. *Movement Dis* 1987; **2**: 1–8.

Tinker R, Anderson MG, Anaud P, Kermode A, Harding AE. Pontine myelinolysis presenting with acute parkinsonism as a sequel of corrected hyponatremia. *J Neurol Neurosurg Psychiat* 1990; **53**: 87–9.

Tolosa ES, Santamaria J. Parkinsonism and basal ganglia infarcts. *Neurology* 1984; **34**: 1516–18.

Ward CD, Duvoisin RC, Ince SE, Nutt JG, Eldridge R, Calne DB. Parkinson's disease in 65 pairs of twins and in a set of quadruplets. *Neurology* 1983; **33**: 815–24.

Weiner WJ, Lang AE. Drug-induced movement disorders (not including tardive dyskinesia). In: *Movement Disorders: a Comprehensive Survey*. Mount Kisco, NY: Futura, 1989: 599–616.

Williams A, Stevenson G, Sturman S, Waring R. Xenobiotic enzyme profiles and Parkinson's disease. *Neurology* 1991; **41** (suppl 2): 29–32.

Wright JJ, Wall RA, Perry TL, and Paty DW. Chronic parkinsonism secondary to intranasal administration of product of meperidine-analogue synthesis. *N Engl J Med* 1984; **310**: 325.

Zhang Z-X, Anderson DW, Mantel N. Geographic patterns of parkinsonism–dementia complex on Guam. *Arch Neurol* 1990; **47**: 1069–74.

Zigmond MJ, Abercrombie ED, Berger TW, Grace AA, Stricker EM. Compensations after lesions of central dopaminergic neurons: some clinical and basic implications. *TINS* 1990; **13**: 290–6.

5
Drug Therapy: General Principles

32. Definitive and symptomatic therapies exist for parkinsonism

Definitive therapy is therapy directed at the pathogenesis of disease, and in the case of parkinsonism, at the cause of the degeneration of dopaminergic cells. Currently, as discussed in maxim 38, most theories of idiopathic parkinsonism postulate neuronal injury induced by free radicals leading to degeneration of dopamine neurons as the cause. Definitive therapy either modifies the production of free radicals or blunts the deleterious effects on the neurons. These therapies will not replace the dopaminergic neurons already destroyed, but are envisioned to slow or halt further neuronal destruction. Thus, definitive therapy should be initiated as soon as the disease is identified or, even better, initiated before symptoms appear if markers for presymptomatic disease become available (Langston, 1990).

Symptomatic therapy, on the other hand, aims to reduce the symptoms of the disease and in parkinsonism is generally directed at augmenting the deficient dopaminergic neurotransmission.

A still theoretical form of therapy – which might be termed reparative therapy – will induce regrowth or replace or substitute other neuronal elements for the destroyed cells. Both tissue grafting and neuronal growth factors hold promise for this form of therapy of parkinsonism (see maxim 100).

33. Initiation of symptomatic therapy depends upon patients' activities and expectations

Symptomatic therapy for parkinsonism should not be automatically started when the diagnosis of parkinsonism is made. Initiation of therapy depends upon the impact of the patient's symptoms on his or her activities. In many patients the diagnosis of parkinsonism may be made when the only symptom is a mild tremor and clumsiness in one hand not materially affecting normal activities. Symptomatic therapy is generally not indicated in this situation. Therapy is initiated when the patient's normal activities are impaired by the disease. Because the onset and progression of the disease are insidious, the patient may not be as aware of the loss of function as are the spouse and close friends. Their perception of the patient's daily functioning should be sought in making the decision to initiate therapy. Thus, the decision to start symptomatic therapy is based more on history than on the examination, although the exam should verify that the patient's signs are consistent with the complaints and that the complaints do not represent problems other than parkinsonism.

The question of when to start therapy is not only complicated by the issues of acute adverse effects, cost, and convenience – which attend all decisions about drug therapy – but also by the concern that the duration of levodopa therapy is proportional to the incidence of the major adverse effects of chronic levodopa therapy; i.e. the fluctuating response and dyskinesia (Fahn and Calne, 1978; Fahn and Bresman, 1984; Duvoisin, 1987). Early initiation of levodopa might then mean that these complications appear earlier and will be present for a greater portion of the patient's life. Furthermore, some believe that long-term therapy causes a loss of efficacy, although the evidence for this is slim. Because of these concerns, however, most neurologists await significant disability – significant being defined by the patient and family – before beginning therapy and particularly levodopa therapy. However, there is also evidence to the contrary; i.e. that delaying therapy unnecessarily deprives the patient of improved motor function during the early course of the disease (Markham and Diamond, 1981) and increases mortality (Diamond et al., 1987).

An effort to delay levodopa therapy as long as possible can be detrimental to the patient if carried to extreme. The patient should not be deprived of the benefits of levodopa if he has significant disability, nor should the patient be administered a vast array of other drugs in an attempt to avoid levodopa. Finally, the use of levodopa should not be portrayed to the patient as the final, desperate means to treat the disease; levodopa is our most efficacious antiparkinsonian drug which benefits most patients for many years.

34.   Tailor symptomatic drug therapy to the patient's symptoms and other neurological and medical problems

The first step in selecting the appropriate drug is for the patient and physician to agree on therapeutic targets. Treating symptoms which are of no importance to the patient will lead to no benefit for the patient. Drug therapy is directed by the constellation of symptoms and concurrent medi-

Table 34.1 Relative indications and contraindications for commonly used antiparkinsonian drugs

Drug	Indication	Contraindication
Anticholinergic	Tremor, sialorrhea, dysphagia	Cognitive impairment Glaucoma Bladder outlet obstruction
Amantadine	Mild bradykinesia	Renal failure
Levodopa	Bradykinesia, postural disturbances	Confusion, hallucinations
Dopamine agonists	Same as levodopa plus complications of levodopa therapy (fluctuations, dyskinesia)	Same as levodopa
Selegiline	Protective therapy Fluctuations in levodopa-treated patients	Confusion, hypotension

cal and neurological problems. Relative indications and contraindications are presented in Table 34.1.

For example, if tremor is the major disability associated with parkinsonism, the drug of choice would probably be an anticholinergic. If the patient presents with bradykinesia and postural instability, levodopa would be indicated. These guidelines are expanded in the maxims on the individual drugs.

35. Start with low doses and increase slowly

'Low and slow' was a phrase introduced to describe the method to start bromocriptine. However, it is appropriate for all the drugs used for treating parkinsonism. 'Low and slow' reduces the side-effects of the drugs and promotes compliance. This may be particularly important in the elderly patient who may be very sensitive to the drugs. Many 'drug failures' are patients who abandon a drug because of side-effects and not because of lack of efficacy. Parkinsonism is a chronic illness and there is no need to try to achieve an immediate therapeutic triumph with drastic changes in drug regimens.

A corollary to the 'low and slow' principle is that only one drug should be introduced or adjusted at a time.

36.   *Antiparkinsonian drugs should not be discontinued abruptly*

The discontinuation of dopaminergic drugs, particularly levodopa, will result in progressive worsening of the parkinsonism over days to weeks (Cotzias *et al.*, 1969; Ogashara *et al.*, 1984). In more severely affected patients, the parkinsonian disability may be much greater than realized and cessation of dopaminergics may precipitate severe rigidity and bradykinesia; the patient may become confined to bed and subject to aspiration and deep vein thrombosis. Deaths have occurred during 'drug holidays' for these reasons. Furthermore, the realization of how severe the underlying parkinsonism really is may be psychologically devastating to the patient. For some patients who undergo withdrawal of dopaminergic drugs, this realization – and not the physical discomfort – is the most disturbing aspect of the process.

Rarely, withdrawal of dopaminergic drugs can precipitate a syndrome of extreme muscular rigidity, fever and disturbed consciousness, the so-called 'neuroleptic malignant syndrome'. This disorder is accompanied by elevation of muscle enzymes and occasionally by frank rhabdomyolysis, leucocytosis and hyperthermia. The syndrome is life-threatening and requires intensive supportive care and reinstitution of dopaminergic therapy (see maxim 96).

The discontinuation of amantadine or anticholinergics, even if the drugs appear to have little benefit to the patient, may also cause a marked worsening of the patient's parkinsonism despite the fact that levodopa is continued or even increased (Hughes *et al.*, 1971; Horrocks *et al.*, 1973; Timberlake and Vance, 1978). This deterioration appears to be a rebound or withdrawal phenomenon; if the patient remains off the amantadine he will eventually return to his baseline functional status (Timberlake and Vance, 1987). In practice, however, many patients will not endure the days or weeks required to regain baseline and will return to the withdrawn drug. Even gradual reduction of amantadine or the anticholinergic may not avoid this rebound worsening. On the other hand, if the physician feels certain drugs are unnecessary, it is worth trying to withdraw them because many patients discontinue amantadine or anticholinergics without difficulty.

37.   *Avoid polypharmacy*

Polypharmacy is common in the treatment of parkinsonism. Because there are a wide variety of drugs available for parkinsonism, it is tempting to add another drug in response to the patient's complaints. Furthermore, the effect of addition of a drug is often difficult to gauge so that drugs are added but rarely discontinued unless obvious adverse effects appear.

Principles to reduce polypharmacy include:

1. Maximize the benefit from each drug before adding another agent. In particular, carefully adjusting the levodopa regimen is more likely to benefit the patient than adding additional drugs.

2. Have a clear indication for adding another drug, and if the target symptom is not helped by the new drug, discontinue it.

3. Consider nonpharmacologic methods to treat symptoms.

4. Periodically try to reduce or discontinue various drugs in the patient's drug regimen, usually one at a time.

The benefits of reducing polypharmacy are an improved sense of well-being (drugs may function as pharmacologic 'wet blankets'), improved cognition, and better compliance because of simpler drug regimens.

References

Cotzias GC, Papavasiliou PS, Gellene R. Modification of parkinsonism: chronic treatment with L-DOPA. *N Engl J Med* 1969; **280**: 337–45.

Diamond SG, Markham CH, Hoehn MM, McDowell FH, Muenter MD. Multicenter study of parkinson mortality with early versus late DOPA treatment. *Ann Neurol* 1987; **22**: 8–12.

Duvoisin RC. To treat early or to treat late. *Ann Neurol* 1987; **22**: 2–3.

Fahn S, Bressman SB. Should levodopa therapy for parkinsonism be started early or late? Evidence against early treatment. *Can J Neurol Sci* 1984; **11**: 200–6.

Fahn S, Calne DB. Considerations in the management of parkinsonism. *Neurology* 1978; **28**: 5–7.

Horrocks PM, Vicary DJ, Rees JE, Parkes JD, Marsden CD. Anticholinergic withdrawal and benzhexol treatment in Parkinson's disease. *J Neurol Neurosurg Psychiat* 1973; **36**: 936–41.

Hughes RC, Polgar JG, Weightman D, Walton JN. Levodopa in parkinsonism: the effects of withdrawal of anticholinergic drugs. *Br Med J* 1971; **2**: 487–91.

Langston JW. Predicting Parkinson's disease. *Neurology* 1990; **40** (suppl 3): 70–4.

Markham CH, Diamond SG. Evidence to support early levodopa therapy in Parkinson's disease. *Neurology* 1981; **31**: 125–31.

Ogasahara S, Nishikawa Y, Takahashi M, *et al.* Dopamine metabolism in the central nervous system after discontinuation of L-DOPA therapy in patients with Parkinson's disease. *J Neurol Sci* 1984; **66**: 151–63.

Timberlake WH, Vance MA. Four-year treatment of patients with parkinsonism using amantadine alone or with levodopa. *Ann Neurol* 1978; **3**: 119–28.

6
Drug Therapy: Protective Therapy

38. Free radicals may be the final common pathway in pathogenesis of dopaminergic neuronal degeneration

Free radicals or reactive oxygen metabolites are being incriminated in the pathogenesis of a variety of human diseases including parkinsonism. The dopaminergic neurons may be particularly susceptible to free radical damage because oxidation of dopamine by monoamine oxidase (MAO) generates hydrogen peroxide (H_2O_2) which can, in turn, generate the very reactive hydroxyl free radical which damages or destroys cells if not scavenged and detoxified (Spina and Cohen, 1989). Furthermore, auto-oxidation of dopamine produces highly reactive quinones which also damage cells. Finally, the generation of free radicals is promoted by the presence of metal ions, especially iron, in high concentrations in the substantia nigra and globus pallidus. Neurons in these nuclei might therefore be subject to oxidative stress (Olanow, 1990).

These observations are the basis for strategies to slow the progression of parkinsonism by reducing the formation of reactive oxidative metabolites or ameliorating their effect on neurons. Inhibition of monoamine oxidase to reduce formation of H_2O_2, reduction of metal ions to reduce metal ion catalyzed free radical formation, and avoidance of drugs which increase catecholamines such as levodopa, are suggested means to reduce oxidative stress of dopaminergic neurons (Olanow, 1990). Of these, only the inhibition of monoamine oxidase is supported by evidence of efficacy in animal models and in humans (Parkinson's Study Group, 1989). Proposed strategies to reduce the damage of free radicals includes (1) augmentation of the enzymatic processes that deactivate free radicals such as superoxide dismutases, catalases and peroxidases, (2) increasing molecules which inactivate free radicals such as glutathione and vitamin C, and (3) enhancing molecular processes which limit or repair free radical damage such as tocopherol (vitamin E) and oxidoreductases (Cotgreave et al., 1988). Vitamin E is also being investigated as a protective agent for parkinsonism.

39.   *Monoamine oxidase B inhibitors are indicated for most otherwise untreated parkinsonian patients*

The rationale for the use of monoamine oxidase inhibitors to reduce the oxidative stress of the dopamine neuron and to slow the progression of the disorder is discussed in maxim 38. Double-blind studies have indicated that the MAO-B inhibitor, selegiline, will prolong the time from diagnosis to time of treatment with levodopa without producing symptomatic improvement (Parkinson's Study Group, 1989). These studies do not prove that degeneration of dopaminergic neurons is slowed by selegiline but are consistent with that hypothesis. To simplify interpretation, these studies were done in patients that were not receiving other antidopaminergic agents. There is no reason to think that if selegiline retarded the progression of the disorder in untreated patients then it would not do the same in patients receiving symptomatic treatment as well.

Although not conclusive (and, in fact, controversial) the clinical evidence that MAO-B inhibitors alter the progression of parkinsonism is sufficiently compelling that the drugs are indicated for most patients. In practice, we are more enthusiastic about using the drugs in young patients and in newly diagnosed patients who are otherwise untreated.

Which patients should *not* receive MAO-B inhibitors? Patients who are confused are likely to develop more confusion on MAO-B inhibitors. Patients with orthostatic hypotension may have this problem exacerbated by MAO-B inhibitors. Patients with continued nausea with dopaminergic agents may have exacerbation of anorexia and nausea. Finally, in patients with the 'parkinsonism plus' syndromes, in which the pathology involves more than just dopaminergic neurons, MAO-B inhibitors are less likely to retard the disease process, although this has not been explicitly tested.

40.   *Selegiline does not cause hypertensive crises*

Used at the recommended dosage of 10 mg per day, selegiline is a selective MAO-B inhibitor and does not cause hypertensive crises that may occur with the nonselective MAO inhibitors. This is because the uninhibited MAO-A isozyme can metabolize the dietary amines, particularly tyramine, that are responsible for the hypertensive responses. Likewise, selegiline does not potentiate the effects of other sympathomimetic drugs used in cold remedies (ephedrine, etc.) as is common with nonselective MAO inhibitors. Finally, selegiline, unlike nonselective MAO inhibitors, does not cause hypertension when administered with levodopa (Chrisp *et al.*, 1991).

Following the principle of 'low and slow', selegiline is started at one-half of a 5 mg tablet once per day and titrated upward over 1–2 weeks to 5 mg at breakfast and lunch. The drug is administered early in the day to reduce effects on night-time sleep. Doses higher that 10 mg per day do not offer substantially greater clinical benefit; lower doses (2.5 or 5.0 mg) may be effective. Doses greater than 20 mg/day can also inhibit MAO-A so that the adverse effects of nonselective MAO inhibitors become a possibility.

In mildly affected parkinsonian patients who are not receiving symptomatic therapy, selegiline is well tolerated. Orthostatic hypotension can occur and insomnia is reported by a small portion of patients. In more advanced patients who are receiving levodopa and other symptomatic therapy, selegiline may not only cause the problems above, but also may enhance the adverse effects of levodopa and even cause confusion. Reactivation of peptic ulcer disease can occur during selegiline therapy, and so peptic ulcer disease is a relative contraindication to the use of the drug. Selegiline has been reported to cause mild elevations of liver enzymes but only rarely has this elevation been a reason to withdraw the drug (Golbe, 1988; Chrisp *et al.*, 1991).

Two drug interactions are of note. The first and most serious is with pethidine. Delirium and marked muscle rigidity have occurred when pethidine is administered to patients receiving selegiline (Zornberg, 1991). The use of pethidine in selegiline-treated patients is contraindicated and other opiate analgesics should be used with caution. The second, and less well documented, interaction is with fluoxetine. Fluoxetine combined with selegiline may cause hypomania, diaphoresis, peripheral vasoconstriction and hypertension (Suchowersky and de Vries, 1990), although the concomitant use of the two drugs is not yet completely contraindicated.

41.   Selegiline symptomatically benefits the levodopa-treated patient

Selegiline was originally introduced as a symptomatic treatment for parkinsonism on the premise that the inhibition of oxidation of dopamine would potentiate the central actions of levodopa and endogenously formed dopamine. Indeed, selegiline does potentiate the effects of levodopa and often levodopa dosage can be reduced by 10–30%. Predictably it also potentiates the adverse effects of levodopa.

In practice, selegiline is most useful for levodopa-treated patients who are experiencing 'wearing off'. In at least 50% of such patients, selegiline provides a moderate reduction in motor fluctuations by prolonging the effect of each dose of levodopa, thereby reducing the 'wearing off'. The severity of disability when 'off' or the benefit when 'on' is not altered by selegiline. Unfortunately, the benefit from selegiline is often of limited duration; the effect wanes over the first year of treatment. The selegiline can then be withdrawn without any worsening of the clinical condition. Patients with more complex patterns of fluctuations (an 'on–off' pattern) receive little or no symptomatic benefit from the addition of selegiline (Golbe, 1988).

Selegiline usually has little symptomatic effect in patients not receiving levodopa; its main indication is for slowing the progression of the disease (Parkinson's Study Group, 1989). Nevertheless, there are a few patients who undoubtedly improve with selegiline alone.

Despite the drug's effects on MAO, its antidepressant actions appear to be weak and inconsistent (Golbe, 1988). Notwithstanding, some patients receive a significant emotional boost from the drug and a few become hypomanic with it. Most depressed parkinsonian patients, however, are not adequately treated with selegiline alone and require other therapies for their depression.

The major adverse effect of adding selegiline to the regimen of the levodopa-treated patient is increased dyskinesia. This problem may often be handled by decreasing the levodopa dose, but in some patients it is necessary to stop the selegiline. Because not all patients experience increased dyskinesia or a 'levodopa sparing effect', levodopa need not be reduced upon initiation of selegiline; the patient's response to the drug is the key to altering therapy.

Reference

Chrisp P, Mammen GJ, Sorkin EM. Selegiline: a review of its pharmacology, symptomatic benefits and protective potential in Parkinson's disease. *Drugs Aging* 1991; **1**: 228–48.

Cotgreave IA, Moldeus P, Orrenius S. Host biochemical defense mechanisms against prooxidants. *Ann Rev Pharmacol Toxicol* 1988; **28**: 189–212.

Golbe LI. Deprenyl as symptomatic therapy in Parkinson's disease. *Clin Neuropharmacol* 1988; **11**: 387–400.

Olanow CW. Oxidation reactions in Parkinson's disease. *Neurology* 1990; **40** (suppl 3): 32–7.

Parkinson's Study Group. The effect of deprenyl on the progression of disability in early Parkinson's disease. *N Engl J Med* 1989; **321**: 1364–71.

Spina MB, Cohen G. Dopamine turnover and glutathione oxidation: implications for Parkinson's disease. *Proc Natl Acad Sci* 1989; **86**: 1398–400.

Suchowersky A, deVries JD. Interaction of fluoxetine and selegiline. *Canad J Psych* 1990; **35**: 571.

Zornberg GL. Severe adverse interaction between pethidine and selegiline. *Lancet* 1991; **337**: 246.

7
Therapy: Non-Dopaminergic Agents

42. Amantadine produces a modest but transient improvement in bradykinesia

Amantadine hydrochloride was originally introduced as an antiviral agent. Parkinsonian patients taking the drug for prophylaxis against the influenza virus noted a fortuitous improvement in their symptoms, prompting Schwab to test its efficacy in a large uncontrolled trial (Schwab *et al.*, 1969, 1972). Two-thirds of the patients showed improvement on a maximum dose of 100 mg twice a day. One-third of the patients experienced a slow, steady reduction in benefit after 4–8 weeks of treatment, while a more sustained benefit of 3–8 months occurred in the rest.

Subsequent placebo-controlled trials have confirmed amantadine's efficacy, although there has been some disagreement on the duration of benefit and which symptoms are most responsive (Kulisevsky and Tolosa, 1990). In direct comparisons, amantadine is superior to anticholinergics but less effective than levodopa (Parkes *et al.*, 1974). Some studies have noted a declining benefit but eventual stabilization at an improved level, while others have reported sustained improvement in a majority of patients (Parkes *et al.*, 1970; Fahn and Isgreen, 1975). Most studies and clinical experience suggest that amantadine has a similar antiparkinson profile to levodopa (i.e. bradykinesia and rigidity respond better than tremor) but some patients derive a satisfactory reduction in their tremor as well (Obeso and Martinez-Lage, 1987). The effective dose range is small, 100–300 mg/day; for most patients 200 mg/day in divided doses is the maximum effective dose. Increasing the dose above 300 mg/day seldom confers any additional benefit and only increases the risk of side-effects.

Several possible mechanisms of action might explain the efficacy of amantadine for parkinsonism. It appears to have both presynaptic and postsynaptic actions at dopaminergic terminals, suggesting it may have synergistic effects with levodopa (Bailey and Stone, 1975). When levodopa is added to amantadine, as is the usual clinical practice, the amantadine/levodopa combination is no better than placebo/levodopa, but worsening occurs when the amantadine is withdrawn (Parkes *et al.*, 1974). This observation may be misinterpreted as evidence for a continuing beneficial effect of amantadine when in fact it represents a rebound or withdrawal phenomenon. If one waits, the patient generally returns to previous baseline in a few weeks. Nonetheless, occasional patients cannot tolerate the withdrawal of amantadine no matter how long they remain off the drug, indicating a genuine long-term benefit.

Generally no significant additional benefit is derived from adding amantadine to an established optimum dose of levodopa, although some studies have described a modest improvement during the first few months of levodopa treatment (Fahn and Isgreen, 1975). Others have suggested some benefit for motor fluctuations, but the effects are modest (Shannon *et al.*, 1987).

A low incidence of side-effects is one of the major benefits of amantadine and the reason it is sometimes used as adjunctive therapy even though the gain in benefit may be modest. Livedo reticularis and ankle edema are common. Livedo reticularis, a reddish-purple reticular mottling usually limited to the skin of the legs, is generally asymptomatic, and does not require discontinuation of the drug. Only rarely does persistent ankle edema become disabling; it resolves within several weeks after stopping the drug. Much less common, but more troublesome, are the mental side-effects such as confusion, visual hallucinations, depression, insomnia, and nightmares which promptly disappear with discontinuation of the drug. These adverse effects are more apt to occur either in demented or in severely affected patients on multiple drugs. Dry mouth and blurred vision are probably related to anticholinergic properties of amantadine and can modestly potentiate the side-effects of concurrently administered anticholinergics. However, in most studies patients benefited more from the combination of amantadine and anticholinergics than with either agent alone, and with little increase in side-effects (Obeso and Martinez-Lage, 1987). Amantadine is eliminated principally by renal excretion; therefore one must take care when it is given to patients with impairment of renal function.

In summary, amantadine is used primarily as short-term initial monotherapy for 6–12 months for mild to moderate symptoms. A good response can delay the need for Sinemet until further disability appears. Occasionally, patients are adequately controlled for years on amantadine alone. Once levodopa is introduced and the dose stabilized, the amantadine should be tapered and discontinued over a period of weeks, if possible, to avoid polypharmacy. The addition of amantadine to anticholinergics may produce further improvement, but should not be continued if there is no clear-cut benefit for the target symptoms or disability. Whether adding amantadine to Sinemet augments the benefit of Sinemet, particularly in fluctuating patients, is unclear. Dopamine agonists and selegiline are currently used for that purpose; however, because of lower expense and minimal risk of side-effects, a trial of amantadine may be considered.

43.   *Anticholinergics are effective for tremor and sialorrhea*

For a century after the discovery of the efficacy of belladonna alkaloids, anticholinergics were the mainstay of the treatment of parkinsonism. They have been supplanted by levodopa. The mechanism by which anticholinergics act may be to restore balance to a cholinergic–dopaminergic interaction in the striatum, where the dopaminergic deficit leads to overactivity of cholinergic neurons. The role of anticholinergics is now limited to the early treatment of mild symptoms or use as adjunctive therapy for control of tremor and sialorrhea (Comella and Tanner, 1990). These medications were initially felt to improve all signs of parkinsonism equally, but now are considered more effective for tremor and rigidity than for akinesia and postural or gait disturbance (Obeso and Martinez-Lage, 1987). Thus, they are useful for treatment of mild symptoms before the more disabling features of parkinsonism appear, symptoms which require treatment with more potent dopaminergic agents. Tremor is sometimes not satisfactorily controlled by Sinemet or dopamine agonists, and the addition of an anticholinergic can be helpful.

Sialorrhea is actually a misnomer. Drooling is not caused by an excessive production of saliva, but by a reduction in the automatic swallowing and clearing of oral secretions. Sialorrhea is therefore a hypokinetic phenomenon and is more common in the later stages of the disease. Because of their potent effect on akinesia, dopaminergic agents are the most effective treatment, but anticholinergics can be useful for troublesome cases. The effect of anticholinergics on sialorrhea probably depends more on a peripheral action to reduce secretions than on a central action. Therefore, small doses of a peripherally acting anticholinergic with fewer central side-effects (such as propantheline) also may be used. Some patients with swallowing difficulty, however, do seem to respond to small doses of centrally acting anticholinergics when other drugs are ineffective; such medications are worth trying in patients with otherwise drug-resistant dysphagia. A final

Table 43.1 Drugs with central anticholinergic activity

		Usual daily dose range
Anticholinergic	Trihexyphenidyl	2–10 mg
	Benztropine	0.5–4 mg
	Biperiden	4–16 mg
	Procyclidine	5–15 mg
Tricyclic	Cyclobenzaprine	20–40 mg
Antihistamines	Diphenhydramine	25–100 mg
Phenothiazine	Ethopropazine	50–400 mg

indication is for 'off dystonia.' Anticholinergics may reduce levodopa-induced 'off' foot dystonia in some patients (Poewe *et al.*, 1988).

A variety of agents with anticholinergic activity are available (Table 43.1). The most potent and commonly used are the synthetic compounds benztropine mesylate and trihexyphenidyl. Following the rule of 'start low and go slow', benztropine and trihexyphenidyl are started at 0.5 and 1 mg respectively at bedtime and gradually increased to a dosing schedule of two to three times per day and total daily doses of 2 and 6 mg. Although some patients tolerate higher doses of anticholinergics, maximum efficacy generally is seen at these lower doses. Anecdotal evidence suggests that ethopropazine (Parsidol) is better for tremor and has fewer side-effects.

44. *Anticholinergic side-effects are common in the elderly*

The peripheral and central side-effects of anticholinergic drugs are many and are more common in the elderly. Peripheral anticholinergic effects such as dry mouth and impaired accommodation – which causes blurred vision – are almost universal. These complaints generally wane with time and seldom require discontinuation of the drug. More troublesome are constipation, exacerbation of angle-closure glaucoma, and urinary retention; the latter is a special problem in men with prostatic hypertrophy.

The central side-effects of anticholinergic drugs are more disabling and dose-limiting, especially in the elderly, who frequently experience dysphoria, sedation, memory disturbance, delirium and hallucinations at therapeutic doses. In most instances this requires discontinuation of the drug. If the anticholinergic side-effects are not disabling, the physician should gradually taper the drug over weeks to avoid a rebound worsening of the parkinsonism which can be severe and seemingly unresponsive to other dopaminergic agents. If the drug is stopped abruptly, the rebound deterioration can give the false impression that the drug was producing a dramatic benefit. Switching to a lower potency drug may avoid the unwanted side-effect but frequently at the expense of ineffective control of the symptom for which it was given. Because of this array of common side-effects to which the elderly are particularly susceptible, the use of anticholinergics must be carefully considered. The indication should be a symptom that is particularly sensitive to anticholinergic drugs and not just a nonspecific desire to improve the parkinsonism. Anticholinergic side-effects are also commonly seen with many other centrally active drugs – in addition to the antiparkinsonian anticholinergics listed in Table 43.1. Antidepressants, antipsychotics, antihistamines and even peripheral anticholinergics can produce central anticholinergic side-effects.

45.   *Diphenhydramine has weak antiparkinsonian effects but is useful for night-time sedation*

Antihistaminic drugs help the symptoms of parkinsonism through their anticholinergic properties rather than antihistaminic effects. The most commonly used drug of this class, diphenhydramine hydrochloride, has relatively weak anticholinergic properties and correspondingly weak effects on parkinsonian symptoms. It now has virtually no place in the treatment of parkinsonian signs and symptoms.

Antihistaminics produce more sedation than anticholinergics, which limit their usefulness for daytime treatment. However, their sedative effects can be used to advantage at bedtime as a soporific in doses of 25–100 mg. Diphenhydramine has a relatively low propensity to produce confusion or ataxia and is therefore a good drug for the elderly, demented patient who requires temporary sedation or a hypnotic.

References

Bailey EV, Stone TW. The mechanism of action of amantadine in parkisonism: a review. *Arch Int Pharmacodyn* 1975; **216**: 246–62.

Comella CL, Tanner CM. Anticholinergic drugs in the treatment of Parkinson's disease. In: Koller WC, Paulson G (eds), *Therapy of Parkinson's Disease*. New York: Marcel Dekker, 1990: 123–41.

Fahn S, Isgreen WP. Long term evaluation of amantadine and levodopa combination in parkinsonism by double-blind cross-over analyses. *Neurology* 1975; **25**: 695–700.

Kulisevsky J, Tolosa E. Amantadine in Parkinson's disease. In: Koller WC, Paulson G (eds), *Therapy of Parkinson's Disease*. New York: Marcel Dekker, 1990: 143–60.

Obeso JA, Martinez-Lage JM. Anticholinergics and amantadine. In: Koller WC, Paulson G (eds), *Handbook of Parkinson's Disease*. New York: Marcel Dekker, 1987: 309–16.

Parkles JD, Baxter RC, Curzon G. Treatment of Parkinson's disease with amantadine and levodopa. *Lancet* 1970; **1**: 1083–7.

Parkes JD, Baxter RC, Marsden CD, Rees JE. Comparative trial of benzhexol, amantadine and levodopa in the treatment of Parkinson's disease. *J Neurol Neurosurg Psychiatry* 1974; **37**: 422–6.

Poewe WH, Lees AJ, Stern GM. Dystonia in Parkinson's disease: clinical and pharmacological features. *Ann Neurol* 1988; **23**: 73–8.

Schwab RS, England AC, Poskanzer DC, Young RR. Amantadine in the treatment of Parkinson's disease. *JAMA* 1969; **208**: 1168–70.

Schwab RS, Poskanzer DC, England AC, Young RR. Amantadine in Parkinson's disease: review of more than two years of experience. *JAMA* 1972; **222**: 792–5.

Shannon KM, Goetz CG, Carroll VS, Tanner CM, Klawans HL. Amantadine and motor fluctuations in chronic Parkinson's disease. *Clin Neuropharmacol* 1987; **6**: 522–6.

8
Therapy: Levodopa in the Early Stages of Parkinsonism

---

46. *Levodopa, a precursor of dopamine, is the most efficacious treatment for parkinsonism*

Orally administered dopamine is metabolized by the gut and systemically administered dopamine does not reach the brain because the amine does not cross the blood–brain barrier. By these routes, dopamine therefore has no effect on the symptoms of parkinsonism. Precursors of dopamine synthesis are absorbed after oral administration, cross the blood–brain barrier and enhance brain dopamine synthesis.

The synthesis of dopamine in the brain normally begins with the dietary amino acid, tyrosine, which is transported into the brain and thence into catecholaminergic neurons. The amino acid is converted to dihydrophenyl-acetic acid (levodopa) by the enzyme, tyrosine hydroxylase, which is rate limiting in the synthesis of dopamine. When symptoms and signs of parkinsonism appear, striatal tyrosine hydroxylase is reduced to 5–20% of normal. Administration of tyrosine does not appear to affect parkinsonian symptoms, presumably because the depletion of tyrosine hydroxylase limits the ability of tyrosine to enhance dopamine synthesis (Hornykiewicz, 1974).

Administration of levodopa, which is transported into the brain by the same transport system as tyrosine, bypasses this rate limiting step in dopamine synthesis. In the brain, levodopa is decarboxylated by aromatic amino acid decarboxylase (AAAD) to dopamine. Although the decarboxylase is also markedly reduced in the parkinsonian brain, concentrations appear to be adequate to decarboxylate either endogenously or exogenously produced levodopa (Hornykiewicz, 1974).

Orally administered levodopa is extensively decarboxylated to dopamine by AAAD present in the gut, liver, kidney and other tissues. Only an estimated 1% of the administered dose enters the brain. The coadministration of a decarboxylase inhibitor which does not cross the blood–brain barrier reduces the peripheral decarboxylation of levodopa without affecting its conversion to dopamine in the brain. There are two benefits to reducing the peripheral conversion of levodopa to dopamine. First, 75% less levodopa needs to be orally administered. Secondly, inhibiting the conversion of levodopa to dopamine reduces the plasma concentrations of peripheral dopamine, decreasing the side-effects of peripherally generated dopamine. For these reasons levodopa is generally administered in combination with a peripherally active decarboxylase inhibitor: either carbidopa (marketed with levodopa as Sinemet) or benzerazide (marketed with levodopa as Madopar).

An estimated 85% of patients with idiopathic parkinsonism respond to some extent to levodopa. Patients with parkinsonism in which the pathology extends to the striatum and pallidum, such as the 'parkinsonism plus' syndromes, generally respond poorly, if at all to, to levodopa. The failure to respond in these patients is attributed to degeneration of the striatal neuronal targets for dopamine or to degeneration in the output pathways of the basal ganglia. A definite response to levodopa is considered by some investigators to be a criterion for the diagnosis of idiopathic parkinsonism. However, there are autopsy proven examples of typical Lewy body parkinsonism which did not respond to levodopa and, conversely, occasional parkinsonism plus syndromes and parkinsonism secondary to vascular disease or hydrocephalus which did respond to levodopa (Rajput et al., 1990).

The magnitude of improvement in parkinsonism symptoms with levodopa cannot be surpassed, and generally not even equaled, by any other available antiparkinsonian agent. If a patient does not respond to levodopa it is highly unlikely that they will respond to a dopamine agonist. Because levodopa is our most efficacious antiparkinsonian drug, it behoves the physician to maximize the response to levodopa.

47.   Use levodopa in patients with impairment in activities of daily living or decreased employability

Levodopa is indicated in patients with bradykinesia, a symptom which produces impairments in balance and gait, hand dexterity, and oral and written communication. These disabilities interfere with activities of daily living, employment, parenting and other activities important to the patient. Tremor alone is rarely an indication for levodopa. The controversy regarding the initiation of levodopa therapy either early or later in the development of the above disabilities is discussed in maxim 33. In actual practice, however, neurologists in both the 'early' and 'late' camps use the criteria above and generally would initiate levodopa therapy at about the same time in any given patient.

A more difficult question is whether to first try amantadine for disability caused by bradykinesia or to go directly to levodopa. The advantage of using amantadine is that it is modestly effective against these symptoms and therefore the use of levodopa can be delayed (maxim 42). The disadvantage is that amantadine's beneficial effects normally persist for only weeks to months and then levodopa is required to control symptoms. In addition, the amantadine is rarely withdrawn, and the patient is unfortunately then on his or her way to polypharmacy.

Levodopa in combination with a peripheral decarboxylase inhibitor (Sinemet or Madopar) is best begun at a low dose – half of a 100 mg tablet three times per day. Initial administration either with or following meals will reduce gastrointestinal side-effects (see maxims 47 and 49), but within a week or so drug administration should be moved away from meals to enhance absorption. The dose is increased to one tablet three times per day after a week.

48. *Maximum therapeutic benefits of levodopa accrue over weeks*

Levodopa produces both short-duration (hours) and long-duration (days) benefit. Although the short-duration effect is often very subtle in more mildly affected patients who are starting levodopa therapy, some patients will note an improvement in their symptoms with the first dose. This short-duration effect becomes more prominent with chronic therapy; with increasing disease severity this effect results in the fluctuating response ('wearing-off' and 'on–off' phenomena). The long-duration effects of levodopa appear to develop over days to weeks, persisting for days after the drug is withdrawn. Maximum benefit is therefore not realized immediately after starting or adjusting levodopa doses. The short-duration effects are superimposed upon this long-duration effect (Muenter, 1971).

How do these patterns of response to levodopa influence strategy of treatment? Primarily they indicate that titration of levodopa dose upward should be slow such that the patient and the physician can determine the full therapeutic benefit of each dose increment. Generally the patient is maintained on a dose of 100 mg of levodopa (with decarboxylase inhibitor) three or four times per day for several weeks to assess the results of therapy. If a response is present but inadequate, strategies differ. Some clinicians add a dopamine agonist such as bromocriptine or pergolide at this point for the reasons described in maxim 66. If further dopaminergic stimulation is required, however, it is also reasonable to increase levodopa to 600–800 mg/day, given in four doses, before adding a dopamine agonist. The goal is to restore motor function so that the patient can adequately function but not to strive for normality and complete eradication of all signs of the parkinsonism. If no improvement occurs with the levodopa at 300–800 mg/day, the physician should slowly increase the levodopa until improvement appears or toxicity prohibits further increases. Very large doses of 2000–3000 mg/day can often be tolerated and may be required in a rare patient. If the maximum tolerated dose of levodopa yields no response, the addition of a dopamine agonist is unlikely to help the patient.

49. *Anorexia, nausea and vomiting are early, sometimes limiting, side-effects of levodopa*

Gastrointestinal symptoms are a common side-effect of levodopa at the time of therapy initiation. These symptoms are attributed to the peripherally produced dopamine which can activate dopamine receptors in the area postrema of the medulla, an area external to the normal blood–brain barrier. Most patients will experience some anorexia and mild nausea upon beginning levodopa, but these effects rapidly diminish with continued therapy and do not require any intervention. However, in a minority of patients, the nausea may be accompanied by vomiting and attendant weight loss, making it impossible for the patient to tolerate a therapeutic dose of levodopa.

Antiemetics are dopamine antagonists and act by blocking the dopamine receptors of the chemoreceptor trigger zone of the area postrema. If such agents enter the brain, however, they will also antagonize the therapeutic effects of levodopa. The majority of available antiemetics do cross the blood–brain barrier and are thus relatively contraindicated in parkinsonism. The one exception is domperidone, a dopamine agonist which crosses the blood–brain barrier very poorly and is essentially devoid of extrapyramidal side-effects. Currently this drug is available in Europe and Canada but not in the United States. Other peripherally active dopamine antagonists and serotonin 5HT-3 antagonists are under investigation as antiemetics and may prove to be useful in parkinsonism.

Other measures to reduce the gastrointestinal side-effects of levodopa include the following:

1. Start with very low doses of levodopa and titrate upwards very slowly to allow the patient to develop tolerance to the side-effects.

2. Administer levodopa with meals to reduce absorption and high plasma peaks.

3. Use levodopa preparations with the highest ratio of decarboxylase inhibitor to levodopa; for example the 25/100 formulation of Sinemet rather than the 10/100 formulation.

4. Administer extra decarboxylase inhibitor to reduce the generation of peripheral dopamine. Carbidopa (available in the USA as Lodosyn by physician request directly to Merck Sharp and Dohme Pharmaceutical Company) is useful for this purpose.

50. *Dizziness, orthostatic hypotension and cardiac arrhythmias may be early side-effects of levodopa*

Orthostatic hypotension may be present early in treatment but is usually asymptomatic and generally disappears in weeks without limiting the use of levodopa. Orthostatic hypotension may be prominent and symptomatic, however, with the introduction of a dopamine agonist; as with levodopa, fortunately, tolerance to the effect occurs rapidly. These effects are thought to be attributable to central dopaminergic mechanisms in the brainstem cardiovascular regulatory centers. Introduction of the drugs at low doses and with very gradual titration upward over the first weeks of treatment minimizes these symptoms. Patients should be counseled about arising suddenly and how to react to lightheadedness. When orthostatic hypotension appears later in the course of the disease, treatment may be required (see maxim 83).

Dopamine formed from levodopa in the systemic circulation can stimulate cardiac beta-adrenergic receptors to produce cardiac arrhythmias. Although the most common cardiac arrhythmia is an asymptomatic ventricular irritability with extra systoles, more serious tachyarrhythmias may occur. The peripheral decarboxylase inhibitors reduce these adverse effects by reducing the peripheral production of dopamine. Because these effects are believed to be mediated through the beta-adrenergic receptor, propranolol is useful if treatment is warranted. It is important to recognize that arrhythmias are common in the older age group and that arrhythmias should not be attributed to levodopa without investigation and substantiation. If caused by levodopa, they should occur in temporal relation to levodopa dosing (Goldberg and Whitsett, 1971). This can be detected by Holter monitoring (see maxim 86).

Dizziness alone, without vertigo, lightheadedness or orthostatic changes in blood pressure, is a complaint in some levodopa-treated patients for which no cause can be discerned. It may be sufficiently troublesome to prevent the use of the drug.

51. *The response to levodopa is variable, but lack of response requires reassessment of diagnosis and therapy*

Levodopa has a beneficial effect in most patients with parkinsonism. However, not all patients respond to the same extent, and up to 15% of patients do not substantially improve (McDowell *et al.*, 1970; Yahr *et al.*, 1969) (see Table 51.1).

Some of this variation in response is due to the fact that not all features of parkinsonism improve to a similar degree. Of the various signs of parkin-

Table 51.1   Response to six months of levodopa therapy in 100 parkinsonian patients

Percentage improvement	Number of patients
75–100	33
50–74	27
25–49	22
0–24	15
Worsened	3

Source: McDowell (1970)

sonism, bradykinesia and rigidity seem to respond most consistently to levodopa. In the severely affected patient, the effect of levodopa on bradykinesia may be one of the most dramatic therapeutic responses in clinical medicine. Birkmeyer and Hornykiewicz (1961) described, in one of the initial reports of levodopa's beneficial action, the effect of a single intravenous levodopa dose: '. . . briefly suspended or considerably reduced akinesia. Patients who were not able to rise from the horizontal position or to get up when seated managed to accomplish these tasks easily after L-DOPA doses. They walked with normal gestures and were even able to run or jump. The soundless, aphonic speech with indistinct articulation due to palilalia became strong and distinct. For a short time the patients were able to perform motor tasks which were not even approximately accomplished with any other drug.' Although rigidity and bradykinesia are the parkinsonian signs most responsive to levodopa, patients presenting with just rigidity and bradykinesia do not respond as well as those who also have tremor.

Other signs improve less consistently (McDowell *et al.*, 1970; Yahr *et al.*, 1969). Tremor is less often responsive and may only improve after months of treatment. In addition, the response to levodopa varies in different areas of the body. Appendicular symptoms, such as poor hand dexterity or micrographia, tend to improve to a greater extent than axial symptoms such as dysarthria, dysphagia, postural instability, and gait disorders. The lack of response of these latter symptoms to levodopa suggests that they represent damage to nondopaminergic tracts (Bonnet *et al.*, 1987).

Reduction of individual parkinsonian signs does not necessarily translate into better function. In particular, reduction in rigidity does not correlate well with improvement in functional abilities. Induction of side-effects such as hypotension, confusion and hallucinations does not correlate with beneficial response. Levodopa-induced dyskinesia, however, most commonly occurs in patients with an otherwise good response to levodopa.

'Parkinsonism plus' syndromes such as progressive supranuclear palsy or multiple system atrophy generally respond poorly to levodopa, presumably because the pathology in these disorders is not restricted to the substantia nigra; the signs and symptoms of these disorders, therefore, represent more than just dopaminergic denervation. Lack of response to levodopa is one tip-off that one is not dealing with typical idiopathic parkinsonism.

From the discussion above the clinician can predict that the rigid, bradykinetic, tremorous patient will respond better to levodopa than those with parkinsonism plus syndromes or with postural instability. However, in practice levodopa is generally tried in all patients with parkinsonism in whom there are no contraindications because it is still the best drug for treatment of parkinsonism and even modest improvement may be functionally significant to the patient.

For the patient who does not respond to levodopa the physician must consider several possibilities (Table 51.2). First, did the patient receive an adequate trial of levodopa? Often, patients do not receive high enough doses (at least 1000 mg of levodopa with carbidopa per day) for long enough to know whether there was improvement. Curtailment of the trial usually occurs because of gastrointestinal side-effects; reintroducing the drug using the strategies discussed in maxim 49 is often successful. Second, an inappropriate index of improvement – most commonly, tremor – is used by patient and physician. Tremor often does not respond, particularly in the first months of levodopa treatment; bradykinesia, on the other hand, may be substantially better, resulting in improved function. Third, drug interactions may block levodopa's effects. Antiemetics given for levodopa-induced nausea are a common example. Finally, the diagnosis of parkinsonism in a non-responding patient should be re-examined. Does the patient have parkinsonism? Does the patient have a parkinsonism plus syndrome?

Table 51.2   Causes of nonresponse to levodopa

Inadequate levodopa trial
Inappropriate index of response
Drug interactions
Wrong diagnosis

References

Birkmeyer W, Hornykiewicz O. The effect of L-3, 4-dihydroxyphenylalanine (DOPA) on akinesia in Parkinson's syndrome. *Wiener Klinische Wochenschrift* 1961; **73**: 787–8.

Bonnet AM, Loria Y, Saint-Hilaire MH, Lhermitte F, Agid Y. Does long-term aggravation of Parkinson's disease result from nondopaminergic lesions? *Neurology* 1987; **37**: 1539–42.

Goldberg LI, Whitsett TL. Cardiovascular effects of levodopa. *Clin Pharm Ther* 1971; **12**: 376–82.

Hornykiewicz O. The mechanisms of action of L-DOPA in Parkinson's disease. *Life Sci* 1974; 1249–59.

McDowell FH, Lee JE, Swift T, Sweet RD, Ogsbury JS, Kessler JT. Treatment of Parkinson's disease with L-dihydroxyphenylalanine (levodopa). *Ann Inter Med* 1970; **72**: 29–35.

Muenter MD, Tyce GM. L-dopa therapy of Parkinson's disease: plasma L-dopa concentration, therapeutic response, and side effects. *Mayo Clin Proc* 1971; **46**: 231–9.

Parkes JD. Domperidone and Parkinson's disease. *Clin Neuropharm* 1986; **9**: 517–32.

Rajput AH, Rozdilsky B, Rajput A, Ang L. Levodopa efficacy and pathological basis of Parkinson syndrome. *Clin Neuropharm* 1990; **13**: 553–8.

Yahr MD, Duvoisin RC, Schear MJ, Barrett RE, Hoehn MM. Treatment of Parkinsonism with levodopa. *Arch Neurol* 1969; **21**: 343–54.

9
Therapy: Levodopa in Later Stages of the Disease

52. Fluctuations in parkinsonian signs and symptoms occur in untreated patients

Most patients with parkinsonism experience some variation in symptoms throughout the day. The most prominent fluctuations in motor symptoms occur in patients chronically treated with levodopa and are discussed in the next maxim. Nonetheless, variability in parkinsonian motor function occurs without drug treatment, as was well recognized prior to the introduction of levodopa (Fahn, 1981; Marsden *et al.*, 1981) (See Table 52.1).

Freezing refers to the sudden inability to move, most typically while walking. It commonly occurs in patients with moderate or severe bradykinesia and may cause episodes of inability to move the feet for seconds to minutes. Freezing often occurs when the patient is startled, distracted or approaches a doorway or narrow passage. Episodes of freezing may cause the patient to fall forward on to the knees. It may be reduced by levodopa treatment, but sometimes is worsened by high doses of levodopa (Ambani and Van Woert, 1973).

Although stress usually worsens parkinsonism transiently, a sudden improvement in mobility with extreme mental stress or with sudden stimulation may occur and is termed paradoxical kinesis. Oliver Sacks (1990) put it like this: 'Thus one may see such patients, rigid, motionless, seemingly lifeless as statues, abruptly called into normal life and action by some

Table 52.1 Fluctuations in untreated parkinsonism

Freezing
Paradoxical kinesis
Sleep benefit
Transient exacerbation with stress, fatigue, illness
Variability in tremor severity
Exacerbation during menses

sudden exigency which catches their attention (in one famous case, a drowning man was saved by a parkinsonian patient who leapt from his wheelchair into the breakers).'

Improvement in parkinsonian symptoms by nocturnal sleep is reported by patients, who describe that their symptoms are much reduced in the morning, despite having been all night without medication (Marsden, 1980). This effect will last from minutes to hours. Sleep during the day tends not to produce the same effect and some patients awaken from a nap with exacerbation of their parkinsonism. Some untreated patients describe deterioration of motor function in the afternoon; this worsening may be an exaggeration of the normal circadian motor performance cycle.

Tremor may exhibit considerable variation over minutes or hours, depending on limb position, stress and fatigue. It may be voluntarily suppressible for some period of time in the mildly affected patient.

The only biological rhythm recognized to influence parkinsonian symptomatology is the menstrual cycle. Some women of reproductive age report increased parkinsonian symptoms for several days prior to menses (Quinn and Marsden, 1986).

Intercurrent illnesses, often seemingly unimportant, such as a cold, the flu, or shingles, will cause a marked deterioration in the parkinsonism that will outlast the acute illness. Finally, many patients report good days or weeks which cannot be correlated with any obvious external factors.

53. The fluctuating response of treated patients to levodopa has many manifestations

Levodopa-induced fluctuations in various parkinsonian signs and symptoms are rare upon initiation of therapy but become increasingly common with chronic levodopa treatment, eventually affecting 90% of patients treated for ten or more years (Marsden and Parkes, 1977; Fahn, 1974; Barbeau and Roy, 1981).

In general, fluctuations in motor state correlate with the timing of levodopa administration, commonly noticed as the re-emergence of parkinsonian symptoms 2–4 hours after a dose of levodopa – the 'wearing-off' effect (Muenter and Tyce, 1971). In addition to this predictable wearing-off effect, some patients exhibit rapid, seemingly unpredictable swings between mobility (often with dyskinesia) and immobility – the 'on–off' response. These rapid swings add to functional disability; the patient is unwilling to venture outside the home if the ability to walk is unpredictable or if cosmetically or functionally disabling dyskinesia occur.

Although variations in motor symptoms are the most easily recognized types of fluctuations, other symptoms may also exhibit considerable diurnal variability (Table 53.1) and be a cause of disability.

Table 53.1 Levodopa-induced fluctuations

Sign	During periods of levodopa action ('on')	Between periods of levodopa action ('off')
Parkinsonism	Improved	Worsened
Choreoathetosis	Present	Absent
Dystonia	Present	'Off' dystonia
Sensory symptoms	Warmth	Pain, paresthesias
Cognition	Confusion	Confusion, mental slowness
Mood	Normal, euphoria	Depression, anxiety
Autonomic	Diaphoresis, hypotension	Urinary hesitancy, diaphoresis, hypertension,
Respiration	Dyspnoea (respiratory dyskinesia)	Dyspnoea (chest-wall rigidity)

Pain or dysesthesia may fluctuate and parallel the motor function, usually being more prominent during 'off' periods. These sensory symptoms include cramping, aching, stinging, tingling, burning, tightness or tenseness; they may fluctuate as much as motor symptoms and be the most disturbing aspect of parkinsonism (maxim 89).

Fluctuations in mood and cognition are common complaints in patients with parkinsonism treated with levodopa. During 'off' periods, many patients report dysphoria, depression, malaise, lassitude, anxiety, or even panic (Nissenbaum *et al.*, 1987). Conversely, mood generally improves during 'on' periods and may vary from a subjective sense of well-being to frank mania.

The ability to concentrate may vary during the day. In some patients, 'off' periods are accompanied by difficulty in concentration or problem solving, with improvement during 'on' periods. Other patients have the opposite complaints, describing impairment of cognitive abilities during 'on' periods; sometimes these complaints are related to levodopa intoxication (Huber and Paulson, 1990).

A variety of autonomic symptoms may appear in conjunction with the motor fluctuations. Respiratory symptoms may occur during both 'off' and 'on' periods. Some patients may describe dyspnea due to chest wall rigidity during 'off' periods, while other patients may complain of prominent panting or 'air hunger' during 'on' periods (see maxim 84). Urinary hesitancy or retention is a problem during 'off' periods in some patients (maxim 80). Likewise, difficulty with defecation due to anismus (inability to relax the external anal sphincter) can occur during 'off' periods (maxim 86). Excessive sweating can occur as a result of severe dyskinesia, but may also occur in paroxysms during 'off' periods (maxim 83). Blood pressure may fluctuate during both 'on' and 'off' states. Levodopa and dopamine agonists have a hypotensive action, and a mild, asymptomatic drop in blood pressure occurs in most patients following levodopa administration. Some patients, however, may experience symptomatic orthostatic hypotension during 'on' periods, and require specific treatment (see maxim 83). Hypotension during 'on' times may be superseded by hypertension during 'off' periods and could inadvertently lead to a misdiagnosis of essential hypertension if blood pressure were only measured during 'off' periods.

Patients often find it difficult to accurately describe what fluctuates or the relationship of the fluctuations to drug administration. This knowledge is obviously critical to the management of the problem. Observing the patient during one or more dose cycles is very helpful in (1) defining what is fluctuating, (2) developing a common vocabulary for the patient and physician to describe fluctuating signs and symptoms, and (3) designing a treatment strategy.

54.   The development of a fluctuating response is related to the severity of the disease as well as chronic therapy

The severity of parkinsonism and the duration of exposure to levodopa are both important factors in the genesis of motor fluctuations. Motor fluctuations, in general, do not appear with the first few doses of levodopa in patients with Hoehn and Yahr stage II and III disease, the severity of disease at which levodopa is usually started. However, patients with severe parkinsonism (Hoehn and Yahr scale IV and V) at the onset of therapy, such as those with MPTP-induced parkinsonism, exhibit motor fluctuations and dyskinesias within weeks of starting levodopa – as opposed to the months or years for less severely affected patients (Ballard et al., 1985).

One explanation for the relation between disease severity and development of fluctuations is that increasing loss of dopaminergic cells progressively reduces the ability to synthesize, store and release dopamine derived from exogenously supplied levodopa. The result is a shorter response to each dose of levodopa, and in turn, variations in motor function. Several studies support this 'storage' hypothesis. Following levodopa administration to rodents with a nigrostriatal lesion, the peak ipsilateral striatal concentration of dopamine and its metabolite, HVA, are lower and fall more rapidly compared with the unlesioned side (Spencer and Wooten, 1984). Also, in patients with parkinsonism studied by positron emission tomography using F-18 labelled levodopa, the retention of positron signal in the striatum, probably reflecting the storage of F-18 labelled dopamine, is deficient in patients with parkinsonism compared with normal volunteers; further, the retention differs between patients with levodopa-induced fluctuations and those with a stable motor response (Leenders et al., 1986). Finally, the reappearance of parkinsonian symptoms following levodopa infusion has been reported to be more rapid in patients with motor fluctuations than in those with a stable motor response (Fabbrini *et al.*, 1988).

An alternative explanation for the early appearance of motor fluctuations in more severely affected patients is that all levodopa-treated patients fluctuate, but that these fluctuations are only recognized in patients with obvious changes in activities of daily living, gait, dyskinesia, or sensory symptoms. Accordingly, fluctuations would be recognized earlier in the more severely affected patient because of a greater change in motor functioning following levodopa dosing or because of such 'off' symptoms as pain or dystonia. In support of this view, patients without previous levodopa treatment and patients without clinically recognized fluctuations nonetheless exhibit subtle motor fluctuations in bradykinesia during and after a levodopa infusion (Gancher *et al.*, 1988) (see Fig. 54.1).

Chronic levodopa exposure is also important to the emergence of motor fluctuations. The most compelling observation is that neither motor fluctuations nor dyskinesia appear with the first few doses of levodopa, even in the severely affected patients, but take several weeks to develop. If disease severity alone dictated the development of fluctuations and dyskinesia, these symptoms should appear with the first dose of drug. A delay in the onset of levodopa-induced dyskinesia also occurs in monkeys with MPTP-induced parkinsonism (Boyce *et al.*, 1990), suggesting that the response to levodopa somehow changes with continuing exposure to the drug.

We must understand the etiology of fluctuations and dyskinesias to design strategies to minimize or prevent these adverse effects of levodopa. Because of the evidence that chronicity of therapy may play a role, current strategies have emphasized reducing cumulative levodopa exposure by using low doses and also by reducing plasma fluctuations of drug concen-

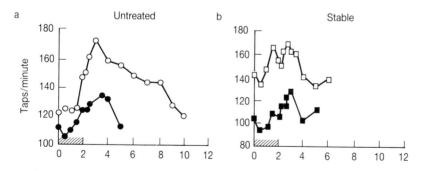

Fig. 54.1 Two patients previously untreated with levodopa (upper) and two reporting a stable response to levodopa (lower) received a 2-hour constant-rate levodopa infusion (shaded area). Each of these 'nonfluctuating' patients exhibited a short-duration response, as measured by performance on a timed task

trations, using controlled release preparations. The success of these strategies has yet to be rigorously proven.

55.   Once the fluctuating response develops, the clinical response to levodopa is dictated by the pharmacokinetic properties of the drug

During the first months or years of levodopa therapy, patients may note little variation in parkinsonism during the day and can omit a dose of levodopa without appreciating any obvious change in symptoms. Eventually, however, most patients begin to note that the beneficial effects of a dose of levodopa fade after two to four hours, serving as a reminder to take the medication. Such patients rarely omit a dose. Even in patients with less clear patterns between levodopa administration and response, an hourly diary of response (on–off chart) averaged over several days may show a relationship between the time of levodopa administration and symptoms; such a relationship may not be apparent when a single day's ratings are examined (Marsden et al., 1981).

These observations suggest a close correlation between plasma levodopa concentrations and clinical effects. The observation that stabilizing plasma levodopa levels by continuous intravenous or enteral infusion markedly lessens fluctuations is further evidence for the importance of plasma levodopa concentrations (Shoulson et al., 1975). Stated another way, motor function in patients with motor fluctuations is dependent upon maintaining plasma levodopa concentrations above some minimal threshold level. The plasma concentrations are determined by the pharmacokinetics of levodopa; the pharmacokinetic properties of levodopa thus determine the clinical response.

The most important pharmacokinetic characteristic of levodopa is its short plasma half-life, approximately one hour (Gancher et al., 1987). This short half-life requires the patient to take multiple daily doses of levodopa to maintain even intermittently effective plasma levels.

Levodopa is prone to significant variation in absorption. It is preferentially absorbed in the small bowel, and factors that slow gastric emptying may delay absorption and affect the clinical response. Failure to absorb a dose of levodopa is a common cause of delayed or absent response to the dose. Variability in absorption of the drug can produce significant alterations in blood levels, because, unlike drugs with a long plasma half-life, sustained blood concentrations are dependent upon constant input or absorption. Food, in particular, may markedly slow absorption (maxim 57). Excessive gastric acidity can cause erratic gastric emptying and slow levodopa absorption; this problem may respond to antacids (Riveracalimlin et al., 1971). Erratic absorption without any obvious cause also occurs (Kurlan *et al.*, 1988).

The transport of levodopa from plasma to brain is another important pharmacokinetic step. Levodopa is transported into the brain by a carrier-dependent saturable transport system, shared by other large, neutral amino acids (LNAAs). High-protein meals elevate plasma LNAA levels, and high concentrations of these other LNAAs can compete for levodopa entry into brain and thereby decrease the clinical response (see maxim 58).

Several strategies which address the short plasma half-life of levodopa have been devised to reduce fluctuations (Table 55.1).

Table 55.1 Strategies used to modify levodopa and dopamine pharmacokinetics to improve response

Treatment	Mechanism	Maxim or reference
Levodopa infusion (intravenous or enteral)	Stabilizes plasma levels	Sage (1988)
Controlled-release levodopa	Prolongs absorption	Cedarbaum (1989)
Low protein meals	Increases transport of levodopa into brain	Maxim 58
Supplemental carbidopa	Decreases peripheral decarboxylation of levodopa	
MAO inhibitors	Reduces dopamine catabolism	Maxims 40, 41
COMT inhibitors	Reduces o-methylation of levodopa and dopamine	

56.   *Unpredictable fluctuations may be iatrogenic*

Patients with unpredictable fluctuations, often referred to as the 'on–off' phenomenon, appear to have random, rapid oscillations in motor state that bear no clear temporal relationship with levodopa dosing (Fahn, 1981; Marsden *et al.*, 1981). The distinction between predictable and unpredictable responses is not absolute, as patients with 'unpredictable' fluctuations still predictably respond to some doses, particularly the first dose of the day. Conversely, patients with 'predictable' fluctuations experience occasional dose failures. The inability to predict the response to each dose of levodopa may be disabling; afflicted patients are unable to plan their daily routines.

There are multiple reasons for apparently 'unpredictable' fluctuations (Table 56.1).

Table 56.1   Causes of unpredictable fluctuations

Frequent, small levodopa doses
Variable absorption
Complex patterns of dyskinesia and dystonia
Lag between levodopa levels and effects

Patients with unpredictable responses are almost always taking multiple small doses of levodopa (Hardie *et al.*, 1984), a common strategy for coping with fluctuations based on the belief that multiple small doses will produce more constant plasma levodopa levels and reduce fluctuations. With a plasma elimination half-life of one hour (Gancher *et al.*, 1988), however, a dose must be taken less than every 30 minutes to maintain a reasonably stable drug level – obviously rarely feasible in practice. Consequently, small frequent doses of levodopa (i.e. every 2–3 hours) do not have the intended effect of stabilizing plasma levodopa levels.

Even worse, there are undesirable consequences of small doses. First, the duration of response is proportional to the dose of levodopa taken, and small levodopa doses produce a briefer response. Secondly, a minimal effective plasma concentration must be reached to gain benefit from levodopa. The smaller the dose, the closer plasma levels will be to this minimum effective concentration, and small variations in absorption may lead to individual doses failing to achieve a clinical effect. Thus the predictable consequence of frequent, small doses of levodopa is unpredictability in clinical response. For this reason, the 'on–off' phenomenon is at least partially iatrogenic, a consequence of dosing schedule.

One treatment strategy that can improve the ability of the patient to predict his or her motor state is to increase the dose and spread out the interval between doses. For example, a patient taking levodopa at two-hour intervals may be unable to predict the response; changing to larger doses of levodopa at 3–4 hour intervals, however, permits predictable improvement in symptoms with each dose. Even if symptoms of parkinsonism re-emerge between doses, the ability to predict motor function may, on the whole, improve daily functioning and allow the patient to plan daily activities, as illustrated by the case report below.

> At age 55, a female patient's complaints of fatigue and left-hand clumsiness were recognized to be parkinsonism; she was begun on levodopa/carbidopa with immediate improvement in her symptoms. She began to note mild dyskinesia and 'wearing off' at age 62, but her levodopa/carbidopa was continued at 200/20 t.i.d. At age 65, her internist became alarmed by asymptomatic blood pressure variations and suggested that she take levodopa/carbidopa 100/10 every 2.5 hours. Not only did she begin to have much more 'off' time, but the beneficial response became unpredictable such that she had to give up driving. Return to a thrice-daily regimen gave her more 'on' time, restored her predictable 'wearing off' pattern and enabled her to resume driving.

The drawback of this strategy may be induction of more severe dyskinesia for longer periods of time.

The pattern of involuntary movements such as dyskinesia and dystonia can confuse the relationship between levodopa dosing and response. Dyskinesia is generally assumed to be the most severe at the peak of levodopa's action, but many patients exhibit diphasic dyskinesias, a pattern in which involuntary movements are more prominent as levodopa's effects begin to wear off (see maxim 59). Peak-dose and 'off' dystonia may be confused, and during the transition between 'on' and 'off' some patients have a mixture of tremor, dyskinesia, and dystonia that defies description. With these complex patterns, it may be difficult for the patient, family or physician to differentiate between these movements or to relate them to timing of doses and presumed blood levels. Some patients are unable to distinguish between dyskinesia and tremor and tend to describe both as 'shaking'.

The clinical effects of levodopa lag behind changes in plasma drug concentrations by 15 to 60 minutes (Shoulson et al., 1975). Because of this lag, administration of levodopa at frequent intervals may obscure the relationship between levodopa administration and clinical response.

57.   Meals affect the response to levodopa

Levodopa is absorbed in the small intestine rather than in the stomach; therefore a slowing of gastric emptying delays drug absorption (Nutt et al., 1984). A number of factors slow gastric emptying, including low gastric pH, anticholinergics, nausea and exercise, but the effect most commonly encountered clinically is of meals. Many patients note that doses of levodopa taken with or immediately after meals may take longer to take effect or may fail altogether. Any food, but particularly those with high fat content, may delay gastric emptying. Although the total amount of drug absorbed after a meal may be similar to that absorbed from an empty stomach, the peak plasma level may be lower and occur later (Fig. 57.1).

Because food delays gastric emptying, it is preferable for patients to take levodopa at least 15–30 minutes *before* meals. If nausea occurs, a light snack (such as fruit, crackers or clear liquids) may lessen the unpleasant feeling. Domperidone, an antiemetic without central antidopaminergic effects, may promote gastric emptying and hasten absorption.

Gastric emptying and consequently levodopa absorption can be accelerated by taking levodopa with warm liquids or with antacids and by chewing the tablets before swallowing. This, in turn, speeds the onset of the clinical effects of levodopa.

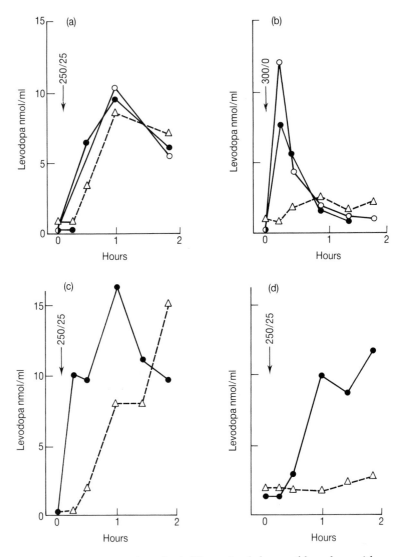

Fig. 57.1 Four patients (panels A–D) received doses of levodopa either on an empty stomach (solid lines) or after a meal (dashed lines). Food delayed or abolished the absorption of levodopa in patients B–D (Nutt *et al.*, 1984)

58. *Manipulation of dietary protein can help some patients*

In addition to slowing levodopa absorption, meals also affect the clinical response to levodopa by affecting the transport of levodopa across the blood–brain barrier. Levodopa crosses the blood–brain barrier by a specific transport mechanism that is shared by the large, neutral amino acids (LNAAs) L-tryptophan, phenylalanine, tyrosine, leucine, isoleucine, and valine. This transport mechanism is saturable, and elevation of the plasma concentrations of these amino acids may competitively inhibit the entry of levodopa into the brain (Fig. 58.1).

As predicted by these observations, high-protein meals may interfere with the action of levodopa, and conversely, low-protein meals may accentuate the effects of levodopa (Nutt *et al.*, 1984; Carter *et al.*, 1989; Tsui *et al.*, 1989; Pincus and Barry, 1987, 1988; Riley and Lang, 1988). A high-carbohydrate meal has the opposite effect. It stimulates insulin secretion

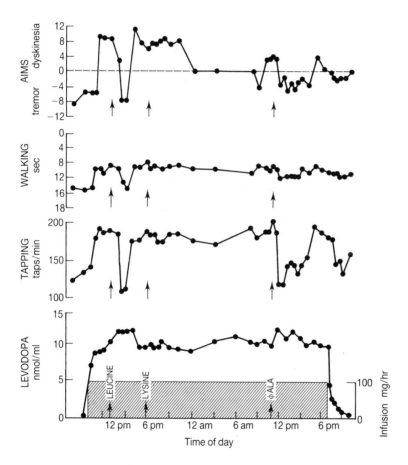

Fig. 58.1 The effects of an oral dose (100 mg/kg) of the large neutral amino acid (LNAA) phenylalanine and the basic amino acid, lysine, in a patient receiving a constant-rate intravenous infusion of levodopa. Motor function did not change following administration of the basic amino acid, but deteriorated following the large amino acid

which promotes transport of LNAAs into muscle and liver and lowers plasma LNAAs – and consequently augments the effects of levodopa (Wurtman, 1990).

The effect of dietary protein on levodopa transport and the clinical state has led to the use of low-protein diets in parkinsonian patients who suffer from fluctuations. Total dietary protein is lowered from the average US intake of 1.6 g/kg per day to the recommended daily allowance of 0.8 g/kg. The protein may be divided equally between three meals, or, in what appears to be an even more clinically effective diet, the 0.8 g/kg is consumed in the evening meal; meals during the day are limited to foods containing little or no proteins, such as fruits and vegetables (Pincus and Barry, 1987, 1988).

Low-protein diets are effective in reducing the 'off' time in patients maintained on the same levodopa dose. In some patients an increase in dyskinesia occurs and requires a lowering the levodopa dose. From what is understood about transport of levodopa into the brain, its entry is proportional to the ratio of plasma levodopa to total plasma LNAA concentrations. Its entry may be increased by increasing the plasma levodopa level (the numerator) or decreasing the plasma LNAA level (the denominator). It is unknown, however, to what extent the effect of reducing protein intake is superior to increasing the levodopa dose.

Low-protein diets are not without adverse effects. They may make difficult the consumption of adequate calories, bran or calcium. Dietary consultation is useful, and the patient's weight should be periodically monitored to detect early malnutrition.

In practice, we use the low-protein diet in fluctuating patients infrequently, choosing those patients in whom other manipulations are unsuccessful for managing their fluctuations and who are capable of following the rather rigorous dietary protocols. Most patients, however, do seem to benefit from simply avoiding foods with very high protein content, and dietary counseling can help them achieve this more limited goal.

59.   A variety of involuntary movements can complicate chronic levodopa therapy

Involuntary movements are unusual with initiation of levodopa therapy, but emerge with chronic treatment. The prevalence of dyskinesia rises to 90% after 10 years of levodopa therapy (Marsden et al., 1981).

The pharmacologic mechanisms underlying levodopa-induced dyskinesias are unknown. Clinical observations suggest that they require (1) dopaminergic denervation, as levodopa does not produce dyskinesias in individuals with normal basal ganglia function, (2) chronic levodopa exposure, as dyskinesias are rare in the newly levodopa-treated patient,

Table 59.1 Levodopa-induced involuntary movements

Manifestations	Temporal patterns
Choreoathetosis	Peak-dose dyskinesia
Dystonia	Diphasic dyskinesia
Ballism	'Off' dystonia
Stereotyped movements	
Myoclonus	
Augmented tremor	
Akathisia	

and (3) intact basal ganglia outflow, as dyskinesias are uncommon in patients who have parkinsonism unrelieved by levodopa (Nutt *et al.*, 1990).

Involuntary movements induced by levodopa may have many manifestations and several temporal patterns (Table 59.1).

Choreoathetosis
The most common levodopa-induced dyskinesia is choreoathetosis, which may involve the face, neck, trunk, extremities, or respiratory muscles. The severity of these movements ranges from subtle – giving an appearance of restlessness – to wild and ballistic.

Levodopa-induced choreoathetosis occurs in two distinct temporal patterns in relation to levodopa administration. The more common pattern is termed 'peak-dose' dyskinesia, in which choreoathetotic movements occur concomitantly with maximum improvement in parkinsonism. The 'peak-dose' term, however, is a bit misleading as it implies that the dyskinesias occur only at the peak action of levodopa (i.e. from one to three hours after levodopa administration) and that periods of improvement in parkinsonism may precede and follow the time that dyskinesias occur. This also suggests that there may be a therapeutic 'window', in which patients may have improvement in parkinsonism without dyskinesia. Although this may occasionally be possible in patients with mild dyskinesias, most patients exhibit dyskinesias throughout the time that the parkinsonism improves (Hardie *et al.*, 1984). In these patients, attempts to lower the levodopa dose to eliminate the dyskinesias usually cause a loss of the therapeutic benefits as well. Therefore, a better term may be 'on dyskinesia', implying the presence of dyskinesias when the antiparkinsonian effects are apparent.

Choreoathetosis may occur in a different pattern, in which chorea signals the beginning and the end of the period of levodopa's action. In most patients with this response, the involuntary movements are more of a mixture of choreoathetosis and dystonia than pure chorea. This pattern has been termed 'diphasic dyskinesia', or the 'D-I-D' response (for dyskinesia–improvement–dyskinesia or dystonia–improvement–dystonia) (Muenter *et al.*, 1977). One interesting pattern of diphasic movements is repetitive foot stamping, kicking, or bicycling movements. These stereotyped movements are distinctive and almost always occur in a diphasic pattern (Marsden *et al.*, 1981; Obeso *et al.*, 1989). It is thought that the involuntary movements occur when the plasma levodopa is at the threshold level.

Dystonia

Dystonia occasionally occurs in untreated parkinsonism (see maxim 89), but is most commonly induced by chronic levodopa therapy. Dystonia occurring with levodopa is similar to idiopathic dystonia, and may involve the upper or lower extremities, face, neck or trunk.

Three distinct temporal patterns of levodopa-induced dystonia are recognized. 'On' or peak-dose dystonia occurs during peak effects of levodopa and is usually admixed with choreoathetosis.

Diphasic dystonia heralds the beginning and the end of a period of levodopa's action and usually lasts only minutes. Like 'on' dystonia, diphasic dystonia usually is admixed with chorea.

Dystonia may also occur as an 'off' symptom and is particularly common in the morning, when the patient has been without levodopa overnight. It disappears as the first dose of levodopa begins to take effect but may reappear with each 'off' period during the day. It especially affects the lower extremities, typically producing inversion and plantar flexion of the foot, but may affect the trunk, neck or upper extremities. In contrast to 'on' or diphasic dystonic movements, 'off' dystonia is usually painful (Melamed, 1979; Nausieda *et al.*, 1980; Poewe *et al.*, 1988).

Treatment of 'on' dyskinesias and of 'on' dystonia are similar. Levodopa dose reduction and adjunctive use of dopamine agonists are helpful in many cases, particularly if the majority of antiparkinsonian action can be achieved with the agonists. However, since many patients have 'on' dystonia or dyskinesia at the same levodopa doses needed to improve parkinsonism, this strategy may not succeed if the agonists alone are insufficient by themselves.

Diphasic choreoathetosis and dystonia appear to occur when plasma levodopa levels enter a window about the threshold for clinical response. Consequently, increasing the size of each levodopa dose causes a more rapid rise in plasma levels and lessens the time that plasma levels are passing through a critical range and keeps plasma levels above the window. This strategy is effective in the short run (L'hermette *et al.*, 1978) but eventually peak-dose dyskinesia or other levodopa toxicity develops, limiting the usefulness of this strategy (Fahn, 1981). Reducing levodopa doses and adding dopaminergic agonists may dampen diphasic dyskinesia.

'Off' dystonia is most prominent in the morning upon first arising. Adjusting night-time doses, using controlled-release preparations, or taking the first dose of levodopa before arising, will reduce 'off' dystonia occurring in the morning. Dopaminergic agonists will often reduce 'off' dystonia.

Discontinuation of levodopa altogether is an option for intractable dyskinesia. All of the above dystonic and choreatic movements disappear with stopping levodopa therapy. This is rarely a permanent solution because of re-emergence of parkinsonism and must be undertaken with great caution (see maxim 60). In some patients, however, adequate mobility can be obtained with the dopamine agonists alone or the dopamine agonists in combination with very small doses of levodopa. Finally, thalamotomy may greatly lessen or eliminate levodopa-induced 'on' dyskinesia and is useful in selected cases when all else fails (see maxim 94). The response of the diphasic dyskinesia and 'off' dystonia to thalamotomy has not been established.

60.   *There are advantages and disadvantages to patient self-titration of Sinemet*

The need for levodopa is not constant from day to day. Many patients find that if they are active they require more levodopa. Likewise, if they are going out for the evening they may need an extra dose of levodopa. On some days, because of dietry or unknown causes, patients seem to require more drug; on other days, however, the dyskinesias may be prominent such that increasing the dose intervals or reducing the size of the doses is appropriate.

The patient who is a good observer may be able to rationally make dose adjustments independently, enabling better control of parkinsonism with fewer side-effects than would be possible when adhering to a rigid levodopa dose schedule. Many times, an optimal levodopa schedule is achieved by trial and error, and it is advantageous for patients to try adjusting their levodopa based on drug response.

On the other hand, there are potential disadvantages to having patients adjust their levodopa. First, it is difficult or impossible for some patients to reliably distinguish between parkinsonism and dyskinesia; the dose adjustments made by these patients may be inappropriate. Second, some drug responses are very confusing and complex, and do not follow simple patterns. For example, a patient with 'off' dystonia and 'on' dyskinesia and dystonia may be unable to determine which specific symptoms are due to recurrent parkinsonism and which are due to acute side-effects of levodopa. Diphasic dyskinesias, in particular, may be very confusing. Third, there is a danger of over-medication with levodopa; some patients may even develop what could reasonably be termed levodopa abuse. Patients with levodopa-induced euphoria or severe 'off' depression or pain are particularly susceptible to escalating levodopa usage and, ultimately, levodopa toxicity.

Thus, the physician must first judge the patient's understanding of fluctuations before allowing the patient to self-titrate levodopa. Second, the physician should establish upper limits to size and number of levodopa doses the patients can take. Self-titration of antiparkinsonian medications other than levodopa is generally ineffective and not necessary. Having the patient keep an 'on–off' chart can establish patterns of response and help the patient increase his or her skill in titrating levodopa.

61. *The role of drug holidays is controversial except in patients with obvious drug toxicity*

A period of levodopa withdrawal (drug holiday) has been advocated to reverse long-term adverse effects that occur with chronic levodopa treatment. Following a 7–10 day drug holiday, levodopa responsiveness appears to be enhanced; lower levodopa doses are needed, and the severity of motor fluctuations, dyskinesia, and psychiatric symptoms are lessened (Weiner *et al.*, 1980; Kaye and Feldman, 1986). Although the mechanism is unclear, some authorities hypothesize that a drug holiday may resensitize dopamine receptors that have been chronically desensitized from exposure to levodopa (however, see maxim 62 below).

The clearest indications for drug holiday are levodopa-induced hallucinations or psychosis that cannot be treated by reducing the levodopa dose or eliminating other drugs. In these patients, levodopa withdrawal may be needed to achieve clearer mentation. Typically, levodopa may then be gradually reintroduced at low doses with fewer side-effects, and this benefit may persist for months.

The role of drug holidays for patients with fluctuations and dyskinesia is arguable (Mayeux *et al.*, 1985). Drug holidays in themselves may have complications and are potentially dangerous. Because the degree of immobility that may ensue is unpredictable, a drug holiday should be undertaken with very close supervision and may require hospitalization. The degree of bradykinesia may be extremely profound, and some patients who are reasonably mobile while treated with levodopa become unable to walk or even turn in bed unassisted. They may develop severe dysphagia, and are at a high risk for a myriad of medical complications including hip fractures, bedsores, aspiration pneumonia, pulmonary emboli, urosepsis, stress ulcers, and neuroleptic malignant syndrome (maxim 96). The severe parkinsonism that is revealed by the holiday is generally much worse than previously experienced and may be psychologically devastating to the patient. In short, drug holidays can be associated with significant morbidity and even mortality.

The long-term efficacy of drug holidays is unclear. Although most patients do exhibit improvement in psychiatric symptoms and motor function soon after the holiday, the improvement gradually wanes over months

(Mayeux *et al.*, 1985). Thus, a drug holiday should be reserved for patients with serious drug toxicity not treatable by other means.

62.   *Patients do not lose their response to levodopa over time*

In the first years of levodopa treatment, the patient may be almost normal when the drug is working. But with continued therapy, most patients are never normal, even at 'optimal' doses of drug; improvement in parkinsonism is marred by dyskinesia or dystonia, and some parkinsonian features fail to improve.

This pattern is often attributed to a 'loss of response'. However, inspection of the degree of response of individual parkinsonian symptoms suggest that such is not the case. Tremor and bradykinesia, common signs in early parkinsonism, continue to respond to levodopa even after 10 years of treatment (Table 62.1). In contrast, postural instability, freezing, dysarthria and dysphagia, symptoms of the later stages of parkinsonism, never respond well to levodopa. Thus, increasing parkinsonian symptoms result from the appearance of levodopa-unresponsive signs, rather than a loss of response of previously responsive signs. A further complication is that dyskinesias, psychiatric side-effects and dementia may obscure improvement in parkinsonism or prevent the administration of effective doses.

The important clinical dictum is that loss of control of a previously levodopa-responsive symptom should not be interpreted as loss of levodopa effect or of disease progression. Instead, the recurrence of symptoms

Table 62.1   Improvement in individual parkinsonian signs over time

Sign	Percent improvement*	
	2 yrs	21 yrs
Tremor	73	85
Rigidity	60	75
Bradykinesia	53	45
Gait	38	28
Postural stability	38	23
Dysarthria	41	24

* Percentage improvement was calculated by rating parkinsonism after withdrawal of levodopa for 1–10 days and after reinstituting treatment (Bonnet *et al.*, 1987).

Table 62.2 Causes of loss of symptom control in parkinsonism

Addition of metaclopramide for GI symptoms
Addition of amoxipine for depression
Addition of neuroleptics for behavioral symptoms
Loss of peristasis from fecal impaction
Noncompliance
Pharmacy error
Intercurrent illnesses
Dehydration and hypotension

---

previously under good control should trigger a search for other treatable etiologies such as drug interactions, difficulties with drug absorption, and intercurrent illnesses (Table 62.2).

63.   Controlled-release levodopa preparations reduce dosing frequency

Two forms of sustained released levodopa have been developed to reduce the fluctuations of plasma levodopa and thereby minimize the fluctuations of motor response to levodopa. Sinemet CR is a slow-eroding matrix containing levodopa and carbidopa which prolongs the absorption of levodopa and thereby produces more sustained plasma levels of drug. Madopar HBS is designed to remain in the stomach, floating on the surface of the gastric contents, and slowly release levodopa and benserazide.

The controlled-release preparations slow the absorption of levodopa so that plasma peaks occur 2–4 hours after drug administration. The consequence is that clinical benefit is delayed. Many patients cannot tolerate the delay, particularly in the morning with the first dose of drug. For this reason many patients are given the controlled-release preparations along with regular preparations of levodopa to shorten the latency to onset of clinical benefit.

Plasma levodopa levels remain elevated longer with controlled-release preparations and therefore dosing intervals can be increased. Patients with uncomplicated fluctuations ('wearing-off') improve because they have a modest reduction in 'off' time. Patients with complicated fluctuations ('on–off') have a less predictable response to controlled-release preparations; in some, the fluctuations are better controlled while in others they are exacerbated. Predicting which patient will benefit is not possible; a trial of the controlled-release preparation is required. Controlled release formulations, particularly Madopar HBS, are helpful for patients with nocturnal akinesia and 'off dystonia'. The use of controlled-release preparations in previously untreated patients is being investigated as a strategy to reduce the development of fluctuations. Controlled-release preparations are clearly effective symptomatic therapy in these patients.

Bioavailability is reduced by 20–30% for Sinemet CR and 40–50% for Madopar HBS. This means that more drug must be given to produce a satisfactory clinical response. Food has less effect on the absorption of the controlled-release preparations than on the regular levodopa formulations, a benefit to patients with erratic absorption.

The adverse effects of controlled-release levodopa are the same as those that occur with regular levodopa. More 'on' time may be associated with more dyskinesia. Likewise, confusion and hallucinations can be exacerbated when the patient is 'on' for longer portions of the day (Marsden et al., 1987; Duvoisin, 1989; Cedarbaum, 1989).

References

Ambani LM, Van Woert MH. Start hesitation – a side effect of long-term levodopa therapy. N Engl J Med 1973; 288: 1113–15.

Ballard PA, Tetrud JW, Langston JW. Permanent human parkinsonism due to 1-methyl-4-phenyl-1,2,3,6-tetrahydropyridine (MPTP): seven cases. Neurology 1985; 35: 949–56.

Barbeau A, Roy M. Ten-year results of treatment with levodopa plus benzerazide in Parkinson's disease. In: Rose FC, Capildeo R (eds), Research Progress in Parkinson's Disease. London: Pitman Medical, 1981: 241–7.

Boyce S, Clarke CE, Luquin R, et al. Induction of chorea and dystonia in Parkinsonian primates. Movement Dis 1990; 5: 3–7.

Carter JH, Nutt JG, Woodward WR, Hatcher LF, Trotman TL. Amount and distribution of dietary protein affects clinical response to levodopa in Parkinson's disease. Neurology 1989; 39: 552–6.

Cedarbaum JM. The promise and limitations of controlled release oral levodopa administration. Clin Neuropharm 1989; 12: 147–66

Christmas TJ, Chapple CR, Lees AJ, et al. Role of subcutaneous apomorphine in parkinsonian voiding dysfunction. Lancet 1988; 2: 1451–3.

Duvoisin RC (ed). New strategies in dopaminergic therapy of Parkinson's disease: the use of a controlled-release formulation. Neurology 1989; 39 (suppl 2): 1–106.

Fabbrini G, Mouradian MM, Juncos JL, Schlegel J, Mohr E, Chase TN. Motor fluctuations in Parkinsons disease: central pathophysiological mechanisms, Part I. Ann Neurol 1988; 24: 366–71.

Fahn S. 'On–off' phenomenon with levodopa therapy in parkinsonism. *Neurology* 1974; **34**: 431–41.

Fahn S. Fluctuations of disability in Parkinson's disease: pathophysiology. In Marsden CD, Fahn S (eds), *Movement Disorders*. London: Butterworth, 1981: 123–45

Gancher ST, Nutt JG, Woodward WR. Peripheral pharmacokinetics of levodopa in untreated, stable, and fluctuating parkinsonian patients. *Neurology* 1987; **37**: 940–4.

Gancher ST, Nutt JG, Woodward W. Response to brief levodopa infusion in parkinsonian patients with and without motor fluctuations. *Neurology* 1988; **38**: 712–16.

Huber SJ, Paulson G. Management of behavioral symptoms in Parkinson's disease. In: Koller WC, Paulson G (eds), *Therapy of Parkinson's Disease*. New York: Marcel Dekker, 1990: 557–6.

Kaye JA, Feldman RG. The role of L-DOPA holiday in the long-term management of Parkinson's disease. *Clin Neuropharm* 1986; **9**: 1–13.

Koller WC, Paulson G (eds). *Therapy in Parkinson's Disease*. New York: Marcel Dekker, 1990: 555–6.

Kurlan R, Rothfield KP, Woodward WR, *et al*. Erratic gastric emptying of levodopa may cause 'random' fluctuations of parkinsonian mobility. *Neurology* 1988; **38**: 419–21.

Leenders KL, Palmer AJ, Quinn N, *et al*. Brain dopamine metabolism in patients with Parkinson's disease measured with positron emission tomography. *J Neurol Neurosurg Psychiat* 1986; **49**: 853–60.

L'hermette F, Agid Y, Signoret JL. Onset and end-of-dose levodopa-induced dyskinesia. *Arch Neurol* 1978; **35**: 261–3.

Marsden CD, Parkes JD. Success and problems of long-term levodopa therapy in Parkinson's disease. *Lancet* 1977; **1**: 345–9.

Marsden CD. On–off phenomenon in Parkinson's disease. In: Rinne UK, Klinger M, Slamm G (eds), *Parkinson's Disease – Current Progress, Problems and Management*. Amsterdam: Elsevier/North Holland, 1980: 241–54.

Marsden CD, Parkes JD, Quinn N. Fluctuations of disability in Parkinson's disease – clinical aspects. In: Marsden CD, Fahn S (eds), *Movement Disorders*. London: Butterworth, 1981: 96–122.

Marsden CD, Rinne UK, Koella WP, Dubuis R (eds). Madopar HBS. International workshop on the 'on–off' phenomenon in Parkinson's disease: new possibilities for its management. *Europ Neurol* 1987; **27** (suppl 1): 1–142.

Mayeux R, Stern Y, Mulvey K, Cote L. Reappraisal of temporary levodopa withdrawal ('drug holiday') in Parkinson's disease. *N Engl J Med* 1985; **313**: 724–33.

Melamed E. Early-morning dystonia: a late side-effect of long-term levodopa therapy in Parkinson's disease. *Arch Neurol* 1979; **36**: 308–10.

Muenter MD, Tyce GM. L-DOPA therapy of Parkinson's disease: plasma L-DOPA concentration, therapeutic response, and side effects. *Mayo Clin Proc* 1971; **46**: 231–9.

Muenter MD, Sharpless NS, Tyce GM, Darley FL. Patterns of dystonia ('I-D-I' and 'D-I-D') in response to L-Dopa therapy for Parkinson's disease. *Mayo Clin Proc* 1977; **52**: 163–74.

Narabayashi H, Yokochi F, Nakajima Y. Levodopa-induced dyskinesia and thalamotomy. *J Neural Neurosurg Psychiat* 1984; **47**: 831–9.

Nausieda PA, Weiner WJ, Klawans HL. Dystonic foot response of parkinsonism. *Arch Neurol* 1980; **37**: 132–6.

Nissenbaum H, Quinn NP, Brown RG, Toone B, Gotham AM, Marsden CD. Mood swings associated with the 'on–off' phenomenon in Parkinson's disease. *Psychol Med* 1987; **17**: 899–904.

Nutt JG, Carter JH. Sensory symptoms in parkinsonism related to central dopaminergic function. *Lancet* 1984; **2**: 456–7.

Nutt JG, Woodward WR, Hammerstad JP, Carter JH, Anderson JL. The 'on–off' phenomenon in Parkinson's disease: relation to levodopa absorption and transport. *N Engl J Med* 1984; **310**: 483–8.

Nutt JG, Carter JH, Woodward WR, Gancher ST. Pharmacodynamics of chronic L-DOPA administration. *Neurology* 1990; **40** (Suppl 1): 292 (abstract).

Obeso JA, Grandas F, Vaamonde J, *et al.* Motor complications associated with chronic levodopa therapy in Parkinson's disease. *Neurology* 1989; **39** (suppl 2): 11–19.

Pincus JH, Barry K. Influence of dietary protein on motor fluctuations in Parkinson's disease. *Arch Neurol* 1987; **44**: 270–2.

Pincus JH, Barry KM. Protein redistribution diet restores motor function in patients with dopa-resistant 'off' periods. *Neurology* 1988; **38**: 481–3.

Poewe WH, Lees AJ, Stern GM. Dystonia in Parkinson's disease: clinical and pharmacological features. *Ann Neurol* 1988; **23**: 73–8.

Quinn NP, Koller W. *Lancet* 1986; **1**: 1366.

Quinn NP, Lang AE, Marsden CD. Painful Parkinson's disease. *Lancet* 1986; **1**: 1366–69.

Quinn NP, Marsden CD. Menstrual-related fluctuations in Parkinson's disease. *Movement Dis* 1986; **1**: 85–7.

Riley D, Lang AE. Practical application of a low-protein diet for Parkinson's disease. *Neurology* 1988; **38**: 1026–31.

Rivera-Calimin L, Dujorne CA, Morgan JP, Lasagna L, Bianchini JR. Absorption and metabolism of L-dopa by the human stomach. *Eur J Clin Invest* 1971; **1**: 313–20.

Sachs O. *Awakenings*. New York: Harper Perennial, 1990.

Sage JI, Trooskin S, Sonsalla PK, Heikkila RE, Duvoisin RC. Long-term duodenal infusion of levodopa for motor fluctuations in parkinsonism. *Ann Neurol* 1988; **24**: 87–9.

Shoulson I, Glaubiger GA, Chase TN. On–off response: clinical and biochemical correlations during oral and intravenous levodopa administration in parkinsonian patients. *Neurology* 1975; **25**: 1144–8.

Snider SR, Fahn S, Isgreen WP, Cote LJ. Primary sensory symptoms in parkinsonism. *Neurology* 1976; **26**: 423–9.

Spencer SE, Wooten GF. Altered pharmacokinetics of L-dopa metabolism in rat striatum deprived of dopaminergic innervation. *Neurology* 1984; **34**: 1105–8.

Tsui JK, Ross S, Poulin K, *et al.* The effect of dietary protein on the efficacy of L-dopa: a double-blind study. *Neurology* 1989; **39**: 549–52.

Weiner WJ, Koller WC, Perlik S, Nausieda PA, Klawans HL. Drug holiday and management of Parkinson's disease. *Neurology* 1980; **30**: 1257–61.

Wutman R, Caballero B, Salzman E. Facilitation of levodopa-induced dyskinesias by dietary carbohydrates. *N Engl J Med* 1988; **319**: 1288–89.

10
Therapy: Dopamine Agonists

64. Dopamine agonists are useful adjuncts to Sinemet

Dopamine agonists are natural or synthetic compounds which directly activate dopamine receptors. The majority are primarily active at the D2 receptor (Table 64.1). Dopamine agonists have several theoretical advantages over levodopa in the treatment of parkinsonism. First, they are not dependent on carrier-mediated transport for absorption or entry into the brain. Their effects will therefore not be influenced by food and plasma amino acids. Second, they do not require metabolic conversion for their dopaminergic activity. Third, some of the dopamine agonists have long plasma half-lives. Fourth, unlike levodopa, they should not generate free radicals when metabolized. Finally, because of a high degree of potency and fat solubility, some of the agonists are well suited for parenteral administration.

The dopamine agonists, particularly apomorphine, are capable of producing an acute antiparkinsonian effect that may equal that of levodopa.

Table 64.1 Properties of dopamine agonists

Agonist	Molecule	Receptor profile	Dose range (mg/day)	Plasma half-life (Hours)	Route
Bromo-criptine	Semisynthetic ergot	D2	15–60	3–7	Oral
Pergolide	Semisynthetic ergo	D1-D2	2–4	24–72	Oral
Lisuride	Semisynthetic ergot	D2	1–4 (1–2)	1–2	Oral, SQ
Apomor-phine	Rearrangement of morphine	D1-D2	(10–100 mg)	30 min	SQ
PHNO	Synthetic	D2	20–60 mg		Oral, SQ Transderm

Sources: Calne *et al.* (1983), Goetz (1990)

In practice, however, only monotherapy in *de novo* parkinsonian patients has been possible. Despite an initial improvement with bromocriptine, pergolide, or lisuride comparable to that of levodopa in *de novo* patients (Riopelle, 1987; Jankovic, 1985), levodopa is almost always eventually needed for an adequate antiparkinson effect (Stern and Lees, 1981). One study of bromocriptine monotherapy in parkinsonism noted that, although 75% of patients were well controlled after one year, more than half needed supplemental levodopa after two years, and eventually almost all patients required levodopa (Rinne, 1985). The reason for this decrement in agonist function is not known; current knowledge about dopamine receptor subtypes and the relative affinities of dopamine and the dopamine agonists does not adequately explain why levodopa is more effective than any of the agonists developed so far. The bottom line, however, is that the dopamine agonists are adjuncts to levodopa therapy.

65. *Dopamine agonists combined with Sinemet may improve control of parkinsonian symptoms in severely affected patients*

Bromocriptine and pergolide may be very valuable as adjunctive treatment of the severely affected patient chronically treated with levodopa. Most levodopa-responsive parkinsonian symptoms improve with the addition of a dopamine agonist because the agonists augment the effects of levodopa. The addition of an agonist is not equivalent to simply adding more levodopa because the agonists have different pharmacokinetic properties and slightly different profiles of benefit and adverse effects, and they are particularly less likely to cause dyskinesias. There is no way, other than trial and error, to determine which patient will benefit from addition of an agonist, but some symptoms are more likely to be helped by agonists (Table 65.1).

The most consistent benefit of adding an agonist is in patients with simple fluctuations ('wearing-off') of response to levodopa. The severity of 'off' periods may be reduced and the duration of the 'on' time increased, smoothing out fluctuations and allowing levodopa to be taken at less frequent intervals. In contrast, patients with poorly predictable fluctuations ('on–off') respond less consistently to the agonists; only a therapeutic trial determines those who will benefit. Nocturnal akinesia (which disrupts sleep) and early morning akinesia – both of which are related to infrequent levodopa dosing during the night – are improved by agonists. Painful 'off' dystonia, in particular, is helped by adding an agonist. Other levodopa-induced dyskinesias, including 'peak-dose' or 'on' choreoathetosis, may be alleviated by adding dopamine agonists and lowering the dose of levodopa. This strategy is particularly effective if the levodopa can be markedly

Table 65.1   Symptomatic response to dopamine agonists in advanced parkinsonism

---

Symptoms amenable to dopamine agonist treament
   Wearing-off response to levodopa
   'Off' or 'early-morning' dystonia
   'Off' pain
   Early morning or nocturnal immobility
   Levodopa-induced dyskinesia (by allowing
      levodopa reduction)
Symptoms less amenable to dopamine agonist treatment
   Unpredictable ('on–off') fluctuations
   Freezing and postural instability
   Poor quality 'on' time
   Lack of response to levodopa
   Diphasic dyskinesias
   Respiratory dyskinesias
   Levodopa-induced hallucinations, psychosis

---

reduced such that the agonist can provide an antiparkinsonian effect that is adequate to keep the patient functional (although this will not be as good as at optimal levodopa effect).

Not all parkinsonian symptoms improve with the addition of a dopamine agonist. In general, dopamine agonists induce a response qualitatively similar to levodopa. Thus, patients with poor or absent response to levodopa do not improve with an agonist and individual signs and symptoms that are resistant to levodopa will not be helped by agonists.

Because dopamine agonists are prone to cause side-effects (see maxim 67), they should be initiated at low doses and the dose increased gradually, taking several weeks to achieve maintenance doses. Bromocriptine, for example, should be started by administering a 1.25 mg dose at night, to lessen the degree of orthostatic hypotension that might otherwise occur if first started during the day. Thereafter, the dose should be incremented by 1.25 mg and later by 2.5 mg every several days, with doses given 3–6 times per day along with the levodopa doses. The bromocriptine dose is increased, as tolerated, to a maintenance dose of 15–40 mg per day; rarely, higher doses, up to 100 mg/day, are used. Pergolide, a drug with approximately 10 times the potency of bromocriptine, should be also started gradually, beginning with 0.125 mg at night and slowly increased. Some patients are poorly tolerant of pergolide, and may require initial doses as low as 0.025 mg. The levodopa dose is not changed upon initiation of dopamine agonists because the initial agonist doses are generally subtherapeutic. As the dose of agonist is increased the physician should watch for augmentation of levodopa's therapeutic and adverse effects and be prepared to reduce the levodopa dose as indicated. Dopamine agonists commonly allow a 20–40% reduction of daily levodopa dose.

Overall, the currently available dopamine agonists improve parkinson-ism to a similar extent and direct comparisons do not indicate that one is superior. However, there are differences in individual patient responses, such that failure to benefit or intolerance to one agonist does not necessarily predict a poor response to another agonist (Goetz *et al.*, 1989; Factor *et al.*, 1988; LeWitt *et al.*, 1983). The benefit to each agonist may wane over months or years (Lieberman *et al.*, 1984); substituting another agonist may restore the response (Goetz *et al.*, 1985).

66.   *The combination of Sinemet and a dopamine agonist at initiation of therapy may reduce long-term side-effects*

The fluctuating response and levodopa-induced dyskinesias appear to be related to the cumulative exposure to levodopa (maxim 53). In order to reduce this exposure, levodopa treatment is customarily delayed until there is a significant degree of motor impairment. Furthermore, the dose of levodopa is kept as low as is possible for adequate, but not full, sympto-matic relief.

One strategy to reduce cumulative levodopa exposure is to use dopamine agonists alone (monotherapy) when the patient first requires dopaminergic stimulation. Though the majority of patients improve to some extent with agonist monotherapy, most patients require the addition of levodopa within months (Rinne, 1987; Goetz, 1990).

Early combinations of levodopa and a dopamine agonist have been recommended as another strategy to minimize the cumulative exposure to levodopa and forestall complications, while providing effective relief of the parkinsonism (Rinne, 1987). Dopamine agonists are used in combi-nation with levodopa initially or are added when low doses of levodopa are inadequate to control symptoms. Most commonly the patient is first started on levodopa; if motor improvement is not sufficient on 300–600 mg of levodopa per day, an agonist is added. This technique is almost always effective in controlling the parkinsonism but the levodopa dose is not much lower than that required to treat symptoms without the added agonist (Rinne, 1987; Factor *et al.*, 1991).

Open studies with a combination of dopamine agonist and levodopa suggest that this strategy is effective in reducing the complications of chronic levodopa therapy (Table 66.1). Preliminary reports of double-blind studies, however, are less clear cut. One such study confirms Rinne's results (described in Goetz, 1990) and another found no advantage of early combination therapy (Factor *et al.*, 1991).

Patients who have not been previously treated with levodopa or who have received the drug for only a short time are more sensitive to orthos-tatic hypotension and gastrointestinal side-effects of the agonists than are

Table 66.1   Prevalence of complications with early combination
bromocriptine–Levodopa (B+L) treatment in Parkinson's Disease

Complication	Levodopa (N=196)	B+L (N=25)
End-of-dose akinesia	67 (34%)	1 (4%)
Early-morning akinesia	46 (24%)	1
Nocturnal akinesia	37 (19%)	1
Freezing episodes, dose-related	38 (19%)	0
Freezing episodes, random	33 (17%)	2 (8%)
Early-morning dystonia	24 (12%)	1
Peak-dose dyskinesia	124 (63%)	6 (24%)

Source: Modified from Rinne (1987)

patients who have been treated chronically with levodopa. The addition of
dopamine agonists to low-dose levodopa during initial therapy, therefore,
should be done gradually, generally starting with bromocriptine doses of
1.25 mg or less and increasing by no more than 2.5 mg per week to doses
of 10–20 mg/day. Pergolide is started at 0.05 mg and slowly increased to
0.5–2 mg/day.

67.   Side-effects of dopamine agonists are similar to levodopa but are more prominent

One of the main difficulties in the use of dopaminergic agonists is the
frequent occurrence of side-effects. Many of the side-effects that occur with
bromocriptine or pergolide are related to dopaminergic stimulation, just as
with levodopa. These side-effects are additive, and decreasing the dose of
either levodopa or dopaminergic agonists will improve the symptoms.
Side-effects of the agonists can be considered in several groups (Table
67.1)

   The first group of adverse effects are probably due to both peripheral
and central dopaminergic effects on blood pressure regulation and gastrointestinal function, producing orthostatic hypotension and gastrointestinal
disturbances. These symptoms are very common in all patients when
therapy is initiated. They tend to abate spontaneously (development of
tolerance?) with continued therapy. Starting with low doses of the agonists
and slowly titrating the dose upwards reduces these side-effects. For
patients with intractable gastrointestinal symptoms, it may be necessary to
add domperidone, an antiemetic without central dopaminergic antagon-
istic actions. The measures discussed in maxim 83 can be used in patients
with persistent orthostatic hypotension.

Table 67.1 Adverse effects of dopamine agonist

Early effects related to central and peripheral dopaminergic mechanisms	Orthostatic hypotension Anorexia, nausea and vomiting
Early or late effects related to central dopaminergic mechanisms	Sleep disturbances and nightmares Depression and agitation Confusion and delirium Hallucinations Psychoses Dyskinesia
Respiratory and cardiovascular toxicity	Dyspnea Pulmonary fibrotic reactions Erythromelalgia Angina Cardiac arrhythmias
Miscellaneous	Reactivation of peptic ulcer disease Dry mouth Headache Nasal stuffiness

The second group of adverse effects, which may occur at any time during treatment with agonists and are consequences of central dopaminergic stimulation, include confusion, hallucinations, psychosis and dyskinesia. These side-effects are more common in patients with severe disease who have been chronically treated with levodopa and who have concomitant dementia. They tend to worsen if the dose of the agonist or of the levodopa is not reduced. Agonist-induced psychosis can be very dramatic and persist for weeks after withdrawal of dopaminergic agents.

The third category of adverse effects of agonists target respiratory and cardiovascular systems and include dopaminergic and idiosyncratic mechanisms. Symptoms may be early or late manifestations of toxicity. Dyspnea may be induced by dopaminergic drugs (see maxim 85) or be related to pulmonary fibrosis. The latter reaction is of uncertain cause but is similar to that described with the ergot alkaloid, methysergide, and it is likely that these drugs share a common mechanism. Erythromelalgia is a painful, red edema of the lower extremities that develops gradually during chronic agonist therapy. Cardiac arrhythmias have not been definitively linked to the dopamine agonists; since they undoubtedly occasionally occur with levodopa, however, it is likely that the agonists can cause similar problems. Angina has also rarely been associated with use of the agonists. This third category of side-effects commonly requires reduction or discontinuation of the agonists.

The final category is a diverse group of adverse effects of uncertain etiology (Table 67.1).

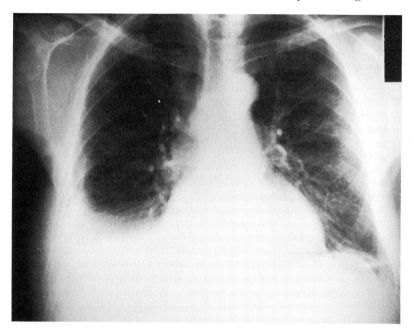

Fig. 67.1 Pleural reaction secondary to dopamine agonist. A 74-year-old man with parkinsonism had been treated with pergolide at doses up to 5 mg/ day for three years when he developed slowly progressive fatigue and short-ness of breath. This chest X-ray revealed obliteration of the right costophrenic angle due to a pleural effusion. Thoracentesis revealed a sterile exudative effusion; pleural biopsies showed nonspecific inflammation and chest and abdominal CT scans were nondiagnostic. Following discontinuation of the pergolide, the pleural effusion and respiratory symptoms resolved after 2–3 weeks

68. *The pharmaceutical properties of dopamine agonists allow parenteral administration*

Patients with motor fluctuations improve when plasma levodopa levels are held constant by intravenous infusion (Hardie *et al.*, 1984; Nutt *et al.*, 1984) or enteral infusion (Cedarbaum *et al.*, 1990; Sage *et al.*, 1988). However, levodopa is difficult to deliver by infusion. The intravenous route is imprac-tical because of (1) the low solubility of levodopa in water, and (2) a tend-ency for levodopa to oxidize in neutral solutions. The enteral route requires enteral access and is cumbersome.

In contrast, several dopamine agonists, including lisuride, apomorphine, and the experimental agonist, PHNO, are well suited for parenteral administration. All are lipophilic, are much more potent than levodopa and are soluble in aqueous solution. These properties allow the agonists to be administered by at least four parenteral routes.

The subcutaneous route is the most commonly employed. Using small, battery-powered ambulatory pumps, apomorphine and lisuride have been given by chronic subcutaneous infusion for 12–24 hours per day for months (Frankel *et al.*, 1990; Stibe *et al.*, 1987; Obeso *et al.*, 1986). Both drugs significantly reduce the need for oral levodopa and apomorphine may even replace levodopa in a few patients. Because apomorphine, unlike lisuride, can fully reverse parkinsonism when injected as a subcutaneous bolus, it has been used as a 'rescue therapy' to reverse 'off' periods that occur during chronic levodopa treatment (Stibe *et al.*, 1988).

Apomorphine has been administered by direct application to a variety of mucous membranes. It is clinically effective sublingually (Lees *et al.*, 1990; Gancher *et al.*, 1990), intranasally (Kapoor *et al.*, 1990) and rectally (Hughes *et al.*, 1991). Although these alternative routes avoid the necessity of self-injection, apomorphine is less well absorbed by these routes than by subcutaneous administration, requiring doses up to 4–6 times higher. The onset of antiparkinsonian effect is also delayed relative to the effect following subcutaneous injection.

Finally, the transdermal route has been used to deliver the experimental agonist, PHNO, from skin patches (Coleman *et al.*, 1989).

Dopamine agonists may also offer another advantage in the future: unlike levodopa, which by conversion to dopamine nonselectively stimulates all dopamine receptors, agonists which more specifically stimulate subpopulations of dopamine receptors may possibly be developed, minimizing some of the side-effects which currently limit levodopa or dopaminergic agonist treatment.

References

Calne DB, Horowski R, McDonald RJ, Wuttke W. *Lisuride and Other Dopamine Agonists*. New York: Raven Press, 1983.

Cederbaum JM, Silvestri M, Kutt H. Sustained enteral administration of levodopa increases and interrupted infusion decreases levodopa dose requirements. *Neurology* 1990; **40**: 995–6.

Coleman RJ, Lange KW, Quinn NP, *et al.* The antiparkinsonian actions and pharmacokinetics of transdermal (+)-4-propyl-9-hydroxynapththoxazine (+PHNO): preliminary results. *Movement Dis* 1989; **4**: 129–38.

Factor SA, Sanchez-Ramos JR, Weiner WJ. Parkinson's disease: an open label trial of pergolide in patients failing bromocriptine therapy. *J Neurol Neurosurg Psychiat* 1988; **51**: 529–33.

Factor SA, Weiner WJ, Sanchez-Ramos J, *et al.* Double blind comparison of bromocriptine and levodopa/carbidopa both alone and in combination in *de novo* parkinsonian patients. *Neurology* 1991; **41** (suppl 1): 172.

Frankel JP, Lees AJ, Kempster PA, Stern GM. Subcutaneous apomorphine in the treatment of Parkinson's disease. *J Neurol Neurosurg Psychiat* 1990; **53**: 96–101.

Gancher ST, Nutt JG, Woodward WR. Sublingual apomorphine in Parkinsons disease. *Movement Dis* 1990; **5** (suppl 1): 53.

Goetz CG, Tanner CM, Glantz RH, Klawans HL. Chronic agonist therapy for Parkinson's disease: a five-year study of bromocriptine and pergolide. *Neurology* 1985; **35**: 749–51.

Goetz CG, Shannon KM, Tanner CM, Carroll VS, Klawans HL. Agonist substitution in advanced Parkinson's disease. *Neurology* 1989; **39**: 1121–2.

Goetz, CG. Dopaminergic agonists in the treatment of Parkinson's disease. *Neurology* 1990; **40** (suppl 1): 50–4.

Hardie RJ, Lees AJ, Stern GM. On–off fluctuations in Parkinson's disease: a clinical and neuropharmacological study. *Brain* 1984; **107**: 487–506.

Hughes AJ, Bishop S, Lees AJ, *et al*. Rectal apomorphine in Parkinson's disease. *Lancet* 1991; **337**: 118.

Jankovic J. Long-term use of dopamine agonists in Parkinson's disease. *Clin Neuropharmacol* 1985; **8**: 131–40.

Kapoor R, Turjanski N, Frankel J, *et al*. Intranasal apomorphine: a new treatment in Parkinson's disease. *J Neurol Neurosurg Psychiat* 1990; **53**: 1015.

Lees AJ, Montastruc JL, Turjanski N, *et al*. Sublingual apomorphine and Parkinson's disease. *Lancet* 1990; **1**: 1440.

Le Witt PA, Larsen TA, Raphaelson MI, *et al*. Comparison of pergolide and bromocriptine therapy in parkinsonism. *Neurology* 1983; **33**: 1009–14.

Lieberman AN, Goldstein M, Liebowitz M, *et al*. Long-term treatment with pergolide: decreased efficacy with time. *Neurology* 1984; **34**: 223–6.

Nutt JG, Woodward WR, Hammerstad JP, Carter JH, Anderson JL. The 'on–off' phenomenon in Parkinson's disease: relation to levodopa absorption and transport. *N Engl J Med* 1984; **310**: 483–8.

Obeso JA, Luqin MR, Martinez-Lage JM. Lisuride infusion pump: a device for the treatment of motor fluctuations. *Lancet* 1986; **1**: 467–70.

Rinne UK. Combined bromocriptine–levodopa therapy early in Parkinson's disease. *Neurology* 1985; **35**: 1196–8.

Rinne UK. Early combination of bromocriptine and levodopa in the treatment of Parkinson's disease: a 5-year follow-up. *Neurology* 1987; **37**: 826–8.

Riopelle RJ. Bromocriptine and the clinical spectrum of Parkinson's disease. *Can J Neurol Sci* 1987; **14**: 455–9.

Sage JI, Trooskin S, Sonsalla PK, Heikkila RE, Duvoisin RC. Long-term duodenal infusion of levodopa for motor fluctuations in parkinsonism. *Ann Neurol* 1988; **24**: 87–9.

Stern GM, Lees AJ. Sustained bromocriptine therapy in previously untreated patients with Parkinson's disease. *J Neurol Neurosurg Psychiat* 1981; **44**: 1020–3.

Stibe CM, Kempster PA, Lees AJ, Stern GM. Subcutaneous apomorphine in parkinsonian on-off oscillations. *Lancet* 1988; **1**: 403–6.

Stibe C, Lees A, Stern G. Subcutaneous infusion of apomorphine and lisuride in the treatment of parkinsonian on–off fluctuations. *Lancet* 1987; **1**: 871.

Vaamonde J, Luquin MR, Obeso JA. Dopaminergic responsiveness to apomorphine after chronic treatment with subcutaneous lisuride infusion in Parkinson's disease. *Movement Dis* 1990; **5**: 260–2.

11
Non-pharmacological Interventions

69. Do not be seduced by drug therapy to the exclusion of other therapeutic modalities

The pharmacological treatment of parkinsonism is rational and effective, characteristics that differentiate the pharmacotherapy of parkinsonism from many other neurologic conditions. It is therefore understandable that the physician equates therapy of parkinsonism with drug therapy and tries to address all complaints with medications. However, some problems are not drug responsive and furthermore, continuing increases in doses or addition of other medications to cope with increasing or new symptoms invariably leads to adverse effects in the elderly. Dependence upon drug therapy to the exclusion of other approaches has another unwanted psychological effect; it places total control and responsibility for treatment on the physician's shoulders and fosters dependency in the patient. Employing non-pharmacological therapies allows patients to have greater participation in their care and a greater feeling of control over their medical destiny.

Non-pharmacologic management requires a different mind-set. The health care provider must assess exactly what is the patient's difficulty, not just make a diagnosis or identify a general problem. Then, a strategy to cope with the specific difficulty must be developed, often requiring innovation which is not guided by much rigorous literature. The care provider must become familiar with community resources to be effective in non-pharmacologic management. These include: physical therapy, occupational therapy, social workers, psychologists, support groups, respite care and local and national lay organizations.

70. *The deterioration in quality of life imposed by parkinsonism may be related more to psychosocial adjustment than to physical disability*

The psychosocial adaptation made by the patient and family to the diagnosis and disability of parkinsonism determines the quality of life. Some patients with minor stigmata of parkinsonism of no functional consequence are psychologically disabled by the threat of progression of physical disability, and other patients with marked physical disability live full, satisfying lives despite the physical limitations. The difference in outcome largely represents psychosocial adjustment. The physician must facilitate this adjustment to manage the patient optimally.

Psychosocial needs change during the course of the disorder. The newly diagnosed or mildly affected patient often harbors unexpressed doubts about the diagnosis, is panicked by the specter of physical and mental deterioration, concerned about cosmetic consequences of parkinsonism, and threatened by employment and financial implications. The physician's role at this point is to educate the patient about how the diagnosis was made and the basic facts about the disorder. The variable progression of parkinsonism and the successful functioning of individuals who have had the disorder for many years is stressed. General support groups are often not helpful at this stage because the support groups invariably contain some severely affected patients who reinforce the mildly affected patient's worst fears. Furthermore, the concerns of general support groups are different from those of the mildly affected person. Support groups that target young or still employed or parenting patients are beneficial if such groups are available. The physician may be able to introduce patients at similar stages of the disease and with similar social and economic backgrounds for one-on-one support. For some patients, a short term of psychological counselling will help them realistically confront the understandably difficult issues of a chronic progressive disease. Financial counselling with a social worker, lawyer or accountant familiar with the issues of chronic disease can aid planning for the future. Joining one or more of the national Parkinson's disease lay organizations (see addresses in the appendix) will keep the patient abreast of research and treatment advances. Finally, the use of drugs believed to slow the progression of the disorder (see maxims 40 and 41), establishing a reasonable exercise program and instituting a generally healthy lifestyle will give the patient a degree of control over his or her disease.

The patient with moderate physical disability must begin to accept limitations without unnecessarily surrendering independence, adapt to changing roles in the family, and appropriately adjust expectations. Group therapy, ideally including patients and spouses, can assist families in this transition. Support groups are very helpful for sharing tricks for coping with physical disability as well as offering psychological support. A number of books and pamphlets supply facts as well as inspiration for coping with parkinsonism (see the appendix). Depression is common and the physician must be alert to its appearance (see maxim 76).

The patient with advanced parkinsonism has markedly impaired mobility and is largely bound to home or an institution, with a consequent shrinking of interaction with other people and decreasing intellectual stimulation. Unfortunately, the spouse assumes greater and greater responsibility for care of the patient and also may withdraw from social interactions. At this stage the physician must help the family draw on community facilities for support, obtain respite care and make the appropriate decisions about nursing home placement. Social workers, nurses, physical therapists and occupational therapists that make home visits are invaluable at this stage to assess and direct medical and psychosocial care.

71.   *Parkinsonism affects the spouse as well as the patient*

Parkinsonism has many implications for the lifestyle of the spouse, affecting living arrangements, retirement and travel plans, financial security, family responsibility and the marital relationship itself. Therefore the spouse not only has a major stake in the successful medical and psychosocial treatment of the patient but is a target for intervention as well. Furthermore the health of the patient is greatly influenced by the medical and emotional health of the spouse.

Common problems for the spouses of parkinsonian patients include: (1) Anger with the patient for the changes in lifestyle caused by his or her illness, often accompanied by guilt for the anger; (2) depression; (3) fatigue, lack of sleep and back strain from demands of caring for the disabled spouse; (4) social isolation as a result of the decreasing mobility of the patient and increasing time required to assist the patient; (5) misunderstanding and misinterpretation of the signs and symptoms of the disease, especially if they fluctuate.

One method to help the spouse is to encourage him or her to accompany the patient to doctor appointments so that they can both express their concerns, learn about parkinsonism and participate in decision making regarding treatment options. Secondly, the spouse should be urged to participate with the patient in support groups or counselling sessions. Thirdly, the physician should remind the patient and spouse that the spouse's health is important to both of them, requiring time apart, maintenance of friendships and outside interests and attention to the spouse's health needs. Fourthly the physician can help the spouse recruit and educate adult children to help care for the patient. Finally, to reduce strife between the marriage partners, the physician should be willing to assume responsibility for unpopular decisions affecting the patient, such as revocation of driving privileges – when a car can no longer be driven safely – and placement in nursing home (Maletta, 1988).

72. *Exercise is important throughout the course of the disease*

Exercise offers many benefits to parkinsonian patients: (1) a sense of well-being; (2) a feeling of control over the disorder; (3) an opportunity for pleasurable interaction with others; (4) improvement of insomnia and constipation; (5) reduction of medical complications of immobility such as venous thrombosis, osteoporosis, atelectasis, contractures and decubiti; and (6) improved general health.

The exercise program must be tailored to the patient's disability and likes and dislikes. The aims of the program should be to maintain full range of motion and strength, and improve mobility, coordination and balance. The program should be enjoyable and safe.

For mild to moderate parkinsonism the exercise program may be that which is appropriate for otherwise healthy individuals of similar age. Walking is excellent. Swimming is also good, although some patients find the synchronization of stroking, kicking and breathing difficult. Patients who freeze while walking may do the same while swimming, sometimes putting them at risk of drowning; adequate supervision of swimming is clearly necessary. A stationary bicycle is good for patients with imbalance. The exercises should not involve activities that would result in serious injury if the patient were to lose balance. Surprisingly, patients often retain well-learned physical skills despite marked rigidity and bradykinesia. Thus the Hoehn and Yahr clinical stage 3 and 4 patient may still play golf, ski, play tennis, dance or play a musical instrument even though activities of daily living are impaired. Timing of medications for optimal motor function during exercise is important for many patients.

At later stages of parkinsonism, the exercise program is best designed by the physical therapist who can evaluate the patient and suggest appropriate stretching and strengthening exercises. National Parkinson's disease organizations also provide excellent exercise booklets and tapes that are appropriate for more advanced patients. Although the goals of exercise are more modest in these patients, exercise helps the patient make full use of their limited physical capacity and continues to give them a sense of well-being and control.

73. *Occupational therapy improves activities of daily living and home safety*

Home evaluation by the occupational therapist is beneficial to the patient with more advanced disease and increasing disability. The therapist can offer techniques and tricks to assist the patient in activities of daily living, particularly dressing, personal hygiene and eating. The therapist can also evaluate the home for safety, particularly assessing floors, stairs, bathrooms and kitchens which account for the majority of home accidents.

Some occupational therapy departments evaluate patients' driving skills, a question that arises during the course of the disease in most patients. The physician may have difficulty evaluating a patient's ability to pilot a car during an office visit, so if doubt exists, assessment by occupational therapy or a driving test with the motor vehicles licensing department should be recommended. In assessing driving capacity, the health care provider should not only be concerned with the patient's motor disability but also the tendency to freeze, the fluctuations in motor function related to levodopa therapy, and insight and judgement (Madeley *et al.*, 1990; Anon, 1990; Dubinsky *et al.*, 1991).

74. *Consider other preventive measures in parkinsonian patients*

The parkinsonian patient with impaired pulmonary function (see maxim 92) is at increased risk for pneumonia and should receive vaccines to prevent pneumococcal pneumonia and the flu. As an aside, any infectious illness, even if mild, often causes a marked deterioration in control of the parkinsonism and the return to pre-illness status may be slow, lagging behind recovery from the infection.

Nutrition is a second concern in the parkinsonian patient. There are many risk factors for malnutrition in this population (Table 74.1).

Table 74.1   Risk factors for malnutrition in parkinsonian patients

Dysphagia secondary to the parkinsonism
Problems with food preparation and feeding
Dementia
Depression
Drug-induced anorexia
Protein and caloric restriction to reduce interference with action of levodopa
Increased caloric requirements because of severe dyskinesia

Body weight is the simplest way in which to follow nutrition. Laboratory indices of malnutrition include: (1) hematocrit and RBC count; (2) total lymphocyte count; (3) serum albumin or transferrin. Improving nutrition in a patient who is unwillingly losing weight will often markedly improve their feeling of general well-being. The indications for a gastrostomy or other feeding tube is discussed in maxim 89. Although the vitamin and calcium needs of the elderly are controversial, it seems prudent to encourage patients to take a multivitamin and supplemental calcium if questions about the adequacy of the diet arise.

75.   Refer patients and families for financial and legal counselling

Chronic neurologic disorders have major financial implications for the patient and family. Loss of employment and the expenses of continuing medical care, adapting the home to the needs of a disabled person, in home care, respite care and nursing home care, are potential threats to the family's finances. Planning for these contingencies requires familiarity with pertinent laws, social security, disability, the many other reimbursement programs for care, insurance and assets and estate planning. Legal issues such as power of attorney, guardianship, joint ownership and trusts become important later in the disease. The health care provider should discretely counsel the patient to confront these issues earlier rather than later in the disease course. To guide the family through this maze one must find a social worker, attorney or financial planner who understands the implications of chronic neurologic disorders and is knowledgeable in the financial and legal issues of providing for families with a disabled person. Support groups for any chronic neurologic disorder, legal aid services or social service departments may be able to provide names of appropriate advisors.

References

Anon. Driving and Parkinson's disease. *Lancet* 1990; **336**: 781.

Dubinsky RM, Gray C, Husted MA, *et al*. Driving in Parkinson's disease. *Neurology* 1991; **41**: 517–20.

Levin BE, Weiner WJ. Psychosocial aspects. In: Koller WC (ed), *Handbook of Parkinson's Disease* New York: Marcel Dekker, 1987: 465–74.

Madeley P, Hulley JL, Wildgust H, Mindhan RH. Parkinson's disease and driving ability. *J Neurol Psych* 1990; **53**: 580–2.

Maletta GJ. Management of behavior problems in elderly patients with Alzheimer's disease and other dementias. *Clin Geriatric Med* 1988; **4**: 719–47.

Nutt JG, Carter JH. Dietary issues in the treatment of parkinsonism. In: Koller WC and Paulson G (eds), *Treatment of Parkinson's Disease*. New York Marcel Dekker, 1990: 531–53.

12
Affective, Cognitive and Sleep Disturbances

76. Mood disorders are common in Parkinson's disease

Depression is common in Parkinson's disease; approximately 50% of the patients suffer from depression at some point in the course of their disease (Mayeux *et al.*, 1984) The disorder may precede the diagnosis of parkinsonism, commonly appears at the time of diagnosis but may also emerge later in the course of the disorder. The severity of the depression is generally mild to moderate, although severe depression with suicide can occur. Depression appears to have at least three etiologies in parkinsonism: reactive, endogenous and drug-induced (Mayeux *et al.*, 1984; Goodwin, 1971).

The diagnosis of depression in parkinsonism may be difficult because many of the vegetative signs of depression may also be manifestations of parkinsonism, including sleep disturbances (maxim 80), sexual disturbances (maxim 82), anorexia, fatigue, and apparent anhedonia (because of facial masking and bradykinesia). There are two particular patterns of depression that are characteristic of parkinsonism. The first pattern is of repeated episodes of depression during the day that correlate with periods when the patient is 'off' (Menza *et al.*, 1990; Nissenbaum, 1987; maxim 53). These 'off' depressive periods may be very distressing, with crying and feelings of complete hopelessness. They are quickly reversed when levodopa again takes effect and for this reason are often interpreted by the patient as being a form of motor fluctuation, as illustrated by the following case.

> A 74-year-old woman who had had parkinsonism for 20 years, initially treated with a right thalamotomy and subsequently with levodopa for 12 years, was referred because of episodes of violent tremor. By history it appeared that the tremor was mixed with dyskinesia and occurred as a 'wearing-off' phenomenon. She was using Sinemet 25/250 four or five times per day, and temazepam 165 mg/day in divided doses to suppress the tremor. The patient was admitted to the clinical research unit for monitoring because of apparent severe motor fluctuations and inappropriate benzodiazepine use.
>
> Monitoring showed that indeed the woman had 'wearing-off' but that the

symptoms were primarily the development of tremor in one leg and were not associated with major motor disability. Her mood, however, changed dramatically between 'on' periods – when she was pleasant and interacted well – and 'off' periods – when she was depressed, anxious, preoccupied with the tremor, and unable to interact meaningfully with other people. Instituting antidepressant therapy and tapering and discontinuing the benzodiazepines improved the patient's overall mood but she still experienced the 'off' depression and anxiety.

A second pattern of depression in parkinsonism is agitated depression with components of panic. This form of depression may also fluctuate during the day (Schiffer et al., 1988).

Treatment of depression is essentially the same as for other elderly patients. The patient's drug regimen should be re-evaluated and any unessential drugs that might contribute to depression (e.g. propranolol, benzodiazepines) discontinued. Occasionally, levodopa or dopamine agonists are responsible for the depression; suspicion is heightened by the temporal coincidence of the onset of the depression with the addition of dopaminergic drugs. Lowering the dose will sometimes improve mood while still benefiting the parkinsonism. Tricyclics, commonly amitriptyline or imipramine, are the mainstays of treatment, generally in doses of 10–75 mg as a single night-time dose. Antidepressants without anticholinergic side-effects are often better tolerated in the elderly, and drugs with alerting or sedating properties may be selected depending upon the patient's anxiety level and sleep behavior (Table 75.1). Nonselective monoamine oxidase inhibitors are contraindicated in levodopa-treated patients because they can cause hypertensive crises. Selective MAO inhibitors such as selegiline are not very effective antidepressants but are generally safe. A possible exception is an interaction between fluoxetine and selegiline, which may produce mania and hypertension (Suchowersky and deVries, 1990). Counselling, encouraging participation in support groups, physical exercise and outside activities improve milder depression. Electroconvulsive therapy can be used in recalcitrant or psychotic depression, often with improvement in the depression and the parkinsonism (Lebensohn and Jenkins, 1975).

Although less common, hypomania occurs in levodopa-treated parkinsonism, and is usually a mild feeling of well-being that accompanies the onset of clinical benefit of each dose, a sensation to which the patient may become addicted. In more marked cases, the hypomania may be manifest by more obvious euphoria with garrulousness, heightened ambition, increased libido and excessive motor activity. Hypomania may also emerge when selegiline is added to the levodopa regimen. As might be expected, hypomania is generally not a source of complaints.

Antidepressants may benefit anxiety as well. If not, small doses of a benzodiazepine such as clonazepam, lorazepam or oxazepam are indicated in some patients – keeping in mind the potential for confusion, ataxia and dependence.

Table 76.1 Characteristics of commonly used antidepressants

Genetic name	Anticholinergic	Sedating	Hypotension	Cardiotoxic
3° amine				
Amitriptyline	+++	+++	+++	+++
Imipramine	++	++	+++	++
2° amine				
Desipramine	+	+	+	++
Nortriptyline	++	++	++	++
Other				
Trazadone	0	+++	+++	+
Fluoxetine	0	0	0	0
Doxepine	++	+++	+++	++

+++ Frequent   ++ Common   + Infrequent   0 Absent

77. *Recognize delirium because it is reversible*

Delirium is characterized by the onset of confusion and altered sensorium over hours to weeks. Orientation, memory and reasoning are impaired. Perception is distorted, producing delusions and hallucinations. Alertness (attention) is either increased, as manifest by agitation or hyperalertness, or is decreased, as evidenced by apathy, abulia, lethargy and somnolence. Distractibility, another manifestation of disturbed attention, is common. Finally, emotional lability, ranging from fear and rage to mania or depression may be present. The patients may exhibit hypo- or hyperactivity (Lipowski, 1989).

The first signs of delirium frequently appear at night as disturbed sleep, confusion, agitation and hallucinations – the so called 'sundowning' syndrome. These signs should therefore trigger a search for reversible causes of confusion. Another characteristic of delirium is for alertness and confusion to fluctuate markedly during the day.

The importance of recognizing delirium is twofold: it is often the first sign of systemic illness in the elderly; and it is generally reversible, i.e. treatable. Although delirium is often superimposed on dementia one should not assume that confusion in the elderly parkinsonian patient is irreversible dementia (Table 77.1).

The differential for delirium is long but can be divided into three general categories. The first is drug-induced. Drugs with anticholinergic properties have been particularly implicated in delirium, but any drug capable of entering the central nervous system – which of course includes all the antiparkinsonian agents and many cardiovascular drugs – can cause delirium. Even some drugs thought to be purely peripherally acting such

Table 77.1   Clinical features differentiating subcortical dementia and delirium

Feature	Subcortical dementia	Delirium
Onset	Months to years	Hours to days
Asterixis, myoclonus, irregular postural tremor	Absent	Present
Attention	Normal, disinterested	Fluctuating hypo- or hyperarousal
Affect	Apathetic, depressed	Fear, suspiciousness, delusional
Perception	Mild disturbances	Prominent visual, auditory hallucinations
EEG	Normal or mild slowing	Marked diffuse slowing

Source: Adapted from Cummings and Benson (1983)

as oxybutynin chloride (Ditropan) can induce delirium. Other drugs, rarely thought of as having central nervous system effects, such as diuretics, cimetidine and nonsteroidals, also are capable of causing delirium (Lipowski, 1989). Withdrawal from alcohol or sedative-hypnotics can produce delirium. Withdrawal from levodopa has even been associated with delirium (Lang, 1987). For these reasons, delirium requires a reappraisal of the patient's drug regimen and an attempt to reduce it to the lowest doses of only the most essential agents.

The second category of etiologies of delirium are systemic illnesses. These may include pneumonia, myocardial infarction, dehydration, electrolyte abnormalities, fecal impaction and congestive heart failure. Surgery frequently precipitates delirium in the parkinsonian patient (Golden *et al.*, 1989). The evaluation of delirium should therefore include a physical exam and laboratory testing for systemic disorders.

The third group of etiologies for delirium are primary neurologic disorders. These include infections of the central nervous system, subdural hematomas, nonconvulsive seizure disorders and, rarely, strokes affecting either the posterior temporal/parietal region or the thalamus. If primary etiologies are serious considerations, the evaluation should include CT or MRI of the brain, EEG and CSF exam.

There are two variants of delirium that are particularly common in parkinsonism. The first is hallucinations, usually visual, of people or animals, occurring without disturbance of sensorium or confusion. The patient may have no difficulty separating the hallucinations from reality. This condition may be stable; it has been termed 'benign hallucinosis'. Unfortunately, these 'benign' hallucinations sometimes progress on to hallucinations that are perceived as real and to paranoid delusions. Hallucinations which occur with a clear sensorium are most commonly associated with dopaminergic treatment and generally respond to lowering or stopping the dopaminergic agents. Because the dopaminergic agonists are particularly potent inducers of hallucinations, they are generally reduced before trying to reduce levodopa. Other antiparkinsonian agents may also contribute to the syndrome and should be discontinued if possible. Short of an emergency, the tapering and discontinuation of drugs should be done systematically, one drug at a time, so that the effects of withdrawal of each drug on the mental status and the parkinsonism can be assessed.

A second variant of delirium seen commonly in levodopa-treated parkinsonism is overt psychosis with paranoia, delusions and hallucinations (again, generally visual). This condition is very frequently associated with dementia or previous mental disorders. Reducing the dopaminergic drugs may improve the psychosis, unfortunately often at the expense of unacceptable worsening of the parkinsonism. The new antipsychotic, clozapine, which has few extrapyramidal side-effects may allow the treatment of the psychosis without exacerbating the parkinsonism (Friedman and Lannon, 1989; Baldessarini and Frankenburg, 1991).

78.   Dementia occurs in 15% of parkinsonian patients

Dementia is characterized by impairment of memory, judgement, abstraction and concentration without alteration in alertness. Dementias may be divided into two categories, cortical and subcortical, based on clinical features (Table 78.1).

Patients with parkinsonism and dementia generally exhibit features of

Table 78.1   Features of cortical and subcortical dementias

Feature	Cortical	Subcortical
Speech	Normal	Dysarthria, hypophonia
Language	Aphasia	Normal
Memory	Amnesia	Forgetful
Reasoning	Impaired, bizarre	Slow, simplistic
Apraxia ⎫ Neglect ⎬ Agnosia ⎭	Present	Absent
Mood	Disinhibited Unconcerned	Apathetic Depressed
Social	Interactive Superficially appropriate	Withdrawn

Source: Adapted from Cummings and Benson (1983)

subcortical dementia, although signs characteristic of cortical dementia may also be present. The physician should not confuse dementia with the slowness of thought, the impaired articulation, bradykinesia and depression that are so common in parkinsonism.

The prevalence of dementia in patients with parkinsonism is controversial (Brown and Marsden, 1987; Gibb, 1989) and is, of course, dependent upon the various criteria of dementia and the population surveyed. All authors agree, however, that the risk of dementia is at least 2–4 times greater in people with parkinsonism than in age-matched controls. The estimated prevalence is 15–20% of the parkinsonian population in most recent studies (Brown and Marsden, 1987; Gibb, 1989).

When confronted with dementia in a parkinsonian patient the physician must consider three etiological categories: (1) other neurologic conditions, (2) drugs and metabolic disorders, and (3) parkinsonism itself and 'parkinsonism plus' syndromes. A routine CBC, chemistry screen, thyroid function, B_{12} and an MRI scan should exclude common metabolic encephalopathies, hypothyroidism, B_{12} deficiency, normal-pressure hydrocephalus, intracranial masses and multi-infarct dementia.

The role of drugs, particularly the antiparkinsonian agents, in the etiology of dementia is often difficult to sort out. Sometimes the patients have an obvious delirium as discussed in maxim 75, and reduction or withdrawal of the drugs will improve mental functioning. Many of these delirious patients will be found to have an underlying dementia, a major risk factor for delirium. However, disturbed attention, the hallmark of delirium, is not present in many parkinsonian patients with impaired cognition. Nevertheless, reduction of unnecessary drugs, particularly any with anticholinergic properties, may improve memory and cognition. If there is no improvement in mental functioning after withdrawal of adjunctive antiparkinsonian medications, a cautious reduction of dopaminergics may be tried, starting with dopaminergic agonists, and weighing the improvement in cognition against the deterioration in parkinsonism.

Neither drugs nor other disorders will be found to explain the dementia in the majority of patients with parkinsonism. Several pathologic bases for the dementia in these patients have been proposed (Gibb, 1989). Many of the patients have pathologic correlates of Alzheimer's disease (Boller *et al.*, 1980). The mesocortical dopaminergic projection is also damaged in parkinsonism, possibly altering cognition (Scatton *et al.*, 1982). The cholinergic neurons of the nucleus of Meynert deteriorate in parkinsonism, possibly contributing to dementia – as is proposed in Alzheimer's disease (Whitehouse *et al.*, 1983). Finally, some demented patients have abundant Lewy bodies throughout the cortex – not just in the substantia nigra compacta. These patients' disorder is termed 'diffuse Lewy body disease' (Bryne *et al.*, 1989; Gibb *et al.*, 1989).

79.   *Behavioral aspects of dementia are manageable*

The behavioral problems, much more than the cognitive deficits, of dementia create problems for family members and caregivers. A number of behavioral disorders occur in demented parkinsonian patients (Table 79.1); importantly, all are to some extent treatable.

The physician should follow a general strategy for managing behavioral problems. First, exclude treatable intercurrent illnesses or avoidable drug adverse effects (in essence, diagnosing and treating delirium [see maxim 77]). Second, consider environmental etiologies for the behavior that might be modified (Table 79.2; Robinson *et al.*, 1988; Winograd and Jarvik, 1986). Third, use behavioral techniques to alter the problem behavior (Table 79.3; Robinson *et al.*, 1988; Winograd and Jarvik, 1986). Alzheimer support groups may be particularly helpful to the family and also provide names of healthcare providers with special expertize in the management of behavioral problems. Fourth, resort to pharmacotherapy when the measures above are not sufficient (Maletta, 1988; Risse and Barnes, 1986; Winograd and Jarvik, 1986). Finally, the physician must realize that management of behavioral problems requires patience and persistence; the problems do not respond to formulas, and trial and error may be necessary to find a successful treatment strategy. Nursing specialists in gerontology and gerontological psychiatrists may be helpful consultants. In addition,

Table 79.1   Common behavioral problems in dementing illnesses

Irrational behaviour
Anxiety and agitation
Bizarre and inappropriate behaviour
Aggressive and assaultative behaviour
Hallucinations, delusions and paranoia
Depression
Wandering
Sleep disorders
Hypersexual behaviour

Table 79.2   Environmental causes of agitation and aggression

Unfamiliar surroundings, people and stimuli
Unfamiliar caregiver
Social isolation
Disrupted daily routine
Inadequate clues to time, place or situation
Overstimulation
Physical restraints
Physical discomfort

Table 79.3   Coping strategies for agitation and aggression

Structure patient's daily routine
Limit stress, decisions, failures
Avoid fatigue and ensure adequate rest
Have patient exercise regularly
Distract patient with other activities when disruptive behavior occurs
Sooth patient with reassuring conversation or physical contact; play
  patient's favorite music
Do not order the patient about; avoid confrontation and argument
Do not expect reasoning to persuade the patient 'to behave'

the caregivers are in great need of support; if they feel abandoned, the patient is soon placed in a nursing home.

Pharmacotherapy of the agitated patient with parkinsonism and dementia is difficult. The class of drugs most commonly used to treat disruptive behavior associated with dementia, the neuroleptics, are relatively contraindicated in parkinsonism because they will – sooner or later – exacerbate the parkinsonism. However, in a few patients the control of the behavior becomes more important than the treatment of the parkinsonism. In this setting a small dose of a neuroleptic with a low incidence of extrapyramidal side-effects may be tried (for example, thioridazine in doses of 25–100mg/day). Attempts to decrease and discontinue the neuroleptic should be made after control of the behavior is achieved. Clozapine, a neuroleptic that is almost devoid of extrapyramidal side-effects, appears very promising for treating psychotic behavior in parkinsonian patients (Friedman and Lannon, 1989; Baldessarini and Frankenburg, 1991).

Benzodiazepines are sometimes successful in reducing agitation. Lorazepam and oxazepam are preferred agents in the elderly because they do not have active metabolites and have half-lives of 8–12 hours. Benzodiazepines may sometimes make behavior worse, intoxicating and disinhibiting the patient. In addition, the benzodiazepines can cause confusion, sedation, amnesia, ataxia and falls in elderly patients. Thus, benzodiazepines should be used sparingly and with careful monitoring in the agitated, demented parkinsonian patient.

The sedating antidepressants without anticholinergic side-effects (for example, desipramine, maprotiline and trazodone) may alleviate nocturnal agitation. Other drugs which occasionally may be helpful in the treatment of agitation and aggression include propranolol, lithium and buspirone (Maletta, 1988; Risse and Barnes, 1986).

The caregiver must be warned that any of these medications can worsen the parkinsonism, the confusion, and even the targeted behavior; the physician must closely monitor the therapeutic and adverse effects.

The caregiver also needs the physician's attention. Depression and 'burnout' are common. The physician must keep in mind the difficulties of the caregiver of a demented individual and offer the caregiver support, education, and access to other community and professional services. The family member who is the caregiver must be encouraged to maintain outside interests and to give themselves time away from the patient. Respite care is essential.

80.   *Sleep disturbances in Parkinson's disease have multiple etiologies*

Disturbed sleep is a common complaint among patients with parkinsonism and, as evidenced by Table 80.1, has many etiologies. Sleep disturbances are often multifactorial with several of the factors identified in the table contributing to poor sleep. The two most common complaints of parkinsonian patients are of multiple awakenings at night and of excessive

Table 80.1   Etiology of sleep disturbances in parkinsonism

Insomnia and sleep fragmentation (nocturnal disruption)	A. Changes with aging
	B. Poor sleep habits
	C. Other sleep disorders
	1. sleep apnea
	2. restless legs
	3. periodic leg movements of sleep (nocturnal myoclonus)
	D. Depression
	E. Parkinson's disease
	1. intrinsic?
	2. rigidity, tremor, pain
	3. cramps and 'off' dystonia
	4. nocturia
	F. Drug-induced
	1. dopaminergic agents
	2. alcohol
	3. sedative hypnotics
	G. Dementia-related
	1. sundowning
	2. day–night reversal
Daytime somnolence	A. Changes with aging
	B. Consequence of nocturnal sleep fragmentation
	C. Drug-induced
	D. Sleep disorders
	1. sleep apnea
	2. narcolepsy

napping during the day. These changes are partially an unavoidable consequence of aging (Prinz et al, 1990) but may be exacerbated by poor sleep habits which are correctable (see Table 80.2).

Other sleep disorders may occur in parkinsonian patients. Sleep apnea is particularly common in multiple system atrophy and may be of either central or peripheral origin; the latter is caused by vocal cord paresis. Restless leg syndrome and periodic leg movements of sleep (nocturnal myoclonus) may often be diagnosed by history; they generally respond to low doses of clonazepam or codeine.

Depression is particularly common in patients with parkinsonism (maxim 76) and sleep disturbance is a common symptom. Treatment with sedating antidepressants such as amitriptyline or trazodone can be immediately effective; antidepressants without sedating effects improve sleep after several weeks of treatment.

Parkinsonism itself may disrupt sleep because of rigidity and bradykinesia. Patients may find it difficult or impossible to roll over in bed or adjust their position and bedding, making them very uncomfortable. Satin sheets, bed rails or a trapeze bar over the bed will help patients with these difficulties. When they awaken during the night, tremor and rigidity reappear and make it difficult to return to sleep. Some patients experience pain as part of the parkinsonism (maxim 92), a serious obstacle to sleep. These nocturnal symptoms of parkinsonism often respond to additional doses of levodopa, generally administered when the patient awakens during the

Table 80.2   Sleep habits

Sleep-wake cycle	1. Establish routine for sleep at night
	2. Promote exercise and social/cognitive activities during the day – not just prior to going to bed
	3. Encourage exposure to bright light, particularly natural (outside) light during the day
	4. Read or develop relaxation techniques for initiating sleep to avoid worrying or problem-solving in bed
Environment	1. Minimize noise and light disruption
	2. Have comfortable bedding and room temperature
	3. Consider problems of sleep partner
	4. Establish bedroom as a place for sleep and peaceful activities
Drug use	1. Limit stimulants such as coffee, tea, soft drinks, tobacco
	2. Limit alcohol in evening which promotes sleep initiation but also causes sleep fragmentation
	3. Avoid chronic use of over-the-counter and prescription hypnotics

Source: Adapted from Prinz et al. (1990)

night. The controlled-release preparations of levodopa, administered as a bedtime dose, appear to be particularly helpful in reducing these problems. Leg cramps and painful 'off dystonia' may interfere with sleep. These problems may respond to extra dopaminergic medications at night, addition of a dopamine agonist to the drug regimen, or to quinine, clonazepam or baclofen at bedtime. Finally, nocturia, whether caused by the 'neurogenic bladder of parkinsonism' or by outlet obstruction, may disturb sleep and may respond to appropriate therapy (maxim 81) with corresponding improvement in sleep.

Dopaminergic drugs alter sleep. Very commonly patients note that their dreams become very vivid. Sleeping partners may describe crying out, jerks or more complex movements during sleep. The symptoms suggest the REM sleep behavior disorder (Schneck et al., 1986; Culebras and Moore, 1989), although polysomnograph recordings indicate that this sleep behavior occurs during slow-wave sleep in parkinsonian patients rather than during REM sleep (Nausieda et al., 1984). The vivid dreaming may be the precursor to hallucinations or delirium and consideration should be given to reducing dopaminergic medications. Small doses of clonazepam at bedtime reduce the REM sleep behavior disorder and may be worth a trial in parkinsonian patients. The dopamine agonists occasionally cause marked insomnia.

The selective MAO-B inhibitor, selegiline, can disturb sleep; for this reason the drug is generally administered as a morning or morning and lunchtime dose to minimize the effects on nocturnal sleep. Even with these measures, some patients must discontinue the drug to obtain a good night's sleep. Conversely, a few patients describe improved sleep with selegiline, perhaps because of increased daytime activity as well as the drug's mild antidepressant action.

Alcohol, over-the-counter hypnotics, and prescribed hypnotics may help induce sleep but increase sleep fragmentation, particularly when used chronically. Furthermore, their use in the elderly is associated with falls (Tinneti et al., 1988), hip fractures (Kay et al., 1987) and diminished alertness and confusion (Morgan, 1990). For these reasons they should be used sparingly for short periods of time, when the titration of antiparkinsonian medications is ineffective. The antihistamine, diphenhydramine hydrochloride, is a mild sleep-inducer that is well tolerated by most patients.

Sleep disturbances often become a major problem in the demented parkinsonian patient. Frequently the patient will have appropriate behavior during the day but become disoriented and hallucinatory at night (sundowning) which keeps the patient awake and promotes nocturnal wandering and other irrational behavior. Consequently the caregiver is also awake and will quickly become exhausted if a solution to the problem or additional help is not provided. The disturbance of nocturnal sleep will generally produce more daytime somnolence; in extreme cases the wake – sleep cycle will be reversed, with the patient sleeping through the day and remaining awake through the night.

Treatment of sundowning is difficult. The basics are to try to promote night-time sleep and reduce daytime sleep by the measures described above for sleep habits. In addition, measures to reduce nocturnal confusion (night lights, familiar surroundings) and to make nocturnal wandering or other activities as safe as possible should be instituted. The drug regimen should be trimmed of all unnecessary drugs, particularly drugs with anticholinergic properties; further dopaminergic agents should be reduced as much as possible without making the patient unbearably parkinsonian. Sedative hypnotic drugs often exacerbate the confusion and may predispose the patient to falls and other injuries. Sedating antidepressants, particularly trazodone, may help. Small doses of antipsychotics such as thioridazine may be necessary but will sooner or later exacerbate the parkinsonism, a price that may be acceptable if the problem is severe. Nocturnal confusion and wandering frequently precipitate placement of the patient in a chronic care facility when the strategy above fails to alleviate the problem.

Daytime somnolence can sometimes be a major problem. Aging, nocturnal sleep fragmentation and, rarely, sleep apnea or narcolepsy may partially explain this symptom. However, most patients relate the somnolence to ingestion of levodopa and to postprandial times which may implicate hypotension as a contributor to the somnolence. The patient commonly describes being unable to sit down to read or watch TV without dozing off; the spouse describes the patient falling asleep during conversations or meals. The physician, however, sees a normally awake patient in the office because this somnolence is generally overcome by any environmental novelty or stimulation. Medical causes of somnolence such as hypotension, anemia, hypercapnia, sedative/hypnotic drugs and subdural hematomas should always be considered in the differential diagnosis of excessive somnolence. Improving nocturnal sleep, reducing levodopa doses and substituting dopamine agonists for levodopa will decrease daytime somnolence in some patients. Stimulants such as caffeine, methylphenidate, pemoline or amphetamine are rarely helpful.

References

Baldessarini RJ, Frankenburg FR. Clozapine: novel antipsychotic agent. *N Engl J Med* 1991; **324**: 746–54.

Boller F, Mitzutani T, Groessman U, *et al.* Parkinson disease, dementia and Alzheimer disease: clinicopathological correlations. *Ann Neurol* 1980; **7**: 329–35.

Brown G, Marsden CD. Neuropsychology and cognitive function in Parkinson's disease. In: Marsden CD, Fahn S (eds), *Movement Disorders 2*. London: Butterworths, 1987: 99–123.

Byrne EJ, Lennox G, Lower J, Godwin-Austin RB. Lewy body disease: clinical features in 15 cases. *J Neurol Neurosurg Psych* 1989; **52**: 709–19

Culebras A, Moore JT. Magnetic resonance findings in REM sleep behavior disorder. *Neurology* 1989; **39**: 1519–23.

Cummings JL, Benson DF. *Dementia: A Clinical Approach*. Boston: Butterworths, 1983.

Friedman JH, Lannon MC. Clozapine in the treatment of psychosis in Parkinson's disease. *Neurology* 1989; **39**: 1219–21.

Gibb WRG. Dementia and Parkinson's disease. *Br J Psychiat* 1989; **154**: 596–614.

Gibb WRG, Luthert PJ, Janota I, Lantos PL. Cortical Lewy body dementia: clinical features and classification. *J Neurol Neurosurg Psychiat* 1989; **52**: 185–92

Golden WE, Lavender RC, Metzer WS. Acute postoperative confusion and hallucinations in Parkinson's disease. *Ann Int Med* 1989; **111**: 218–22.

Goodwin FK. Psychiatric side-effects of levodopa in man. *JAMA* 1971; **218**: 1915–20.

Kay WA, Griffin MR, Schaffner W, Baugh DR, Mellon LJ. Psychotropic drug use and the risk of hip fracture *N Engl J Med* 1987; 316: 363–69

Lang AE. Sudden confusion with levodopa withdrawal. *Movement Dis* 1987; **2**: 223.

Lebensohn ZM, Jenkins RB. Improvement of parkinsonism in depressed patients treated with ECT. *Am J Psychiat* 1975; **132**(3): 283–5.

Lipowski ZJ. Delirium in the elderly patient. *N Engl J Med* 1989; **320**: 578–82.

Maletta GJ. Management of behavior problems in elderly patients with Alzheimer's disease and other dementias. *Clin Ger Med* 1988; **4**: 719–47.

Mayeux R, Williams JBW, Stern Y, Cote L. Depression and Parkinson's disease. *Adv Neurol* 1984; **40**: 241–50.

Menza MA, Sage J, Marshall E, Cody R, Duvoisin R. Mood changes and 'on–off' phenomena in Parkinson's disease. *Movement Dis* 1990; **5**: 148–51.

Morgan K. Hypnotics in the elderly: what cause for concern? *Drugs* 1990; **40**: 688–96.

Nausieda PA, Glantz R, Weber S, Baum R, Klawans HL. Psychiatric complications of levodopa therapy of Parkinson's disease. *Adv Neurol* 1984; **40**: 271–7.

Nissenbaum H, Quinn NP, Brown RG, Toone B, Gotham AM, Marsden CD. Mood swings associated with the 'on–off' phenomenon in Parkinson's disease. *Psychological Med* 1987; **17**: 899–904.

Prinz PN, Vitiello MV, Raskind MA, Thorpy MJ. Geriatrics: sleep disorders and aging. *N Engl J Med* 1990; **323**: 520–6.

Ray WA, Griffin MR, Schaffner W, Baugh DK, Melton LJ. Psychotropic drug use and the risk of hip fracture. *N Engl J Med* 1987; **316**: 363–9.

Risse SC, Barnes R. Pharmacologic treatment of agitation associated with dementia. *JAGS* 1986; **34**: 368–76.

Robinson A, Spencer B, White L. *Understanding Difficult Behaviors: Some Practical Suggestions for Coping with Alzheimer's Disease and Related Illnesses.* Geriatric Education Center of Michigan at Eastern Michigan University, Ypsilanti, MI, 1988.

Scatton B, Rouquier L, Javoy-Agid F, et al. Dopamine deficiency in the cerebral cortex in Parkinson disease. *Neurology* 1982; **32**: 1039–40.

Schiffer RB, Kurlan R, Rubin A, Boer S. Evidence for atypical depression in Parkinson's disease. *Am J Psychiat* 1988; **145**: 1020–2.

Schneck CH, Bundle SR, Ettinger MG, Mahowald MW. Chronic behavioral disorders of human REM sleep: a new category of parasomnia. *Sleep* 1986; **9**: 293–308.

Suchowersky O, deVries JD. Interaction of fluoxetine and selegiline. *Canad J Psychiat* 1990; **35**: 571–2.

Tinetti ME, Speechley M, Ginter SF. Risk factors for falls among elderly persons living in the community. *N Engl J Med* 1988; **319**: 1701–7.

Whitehouse PJ, Hedreen JC, White CL, et al. Basal forebrain neurons in the dementia of Parkinson's disease. *Ann Neurol* 1983; **13**: 243–8.

Winograd CH, Jarvik LF. Physician management of the demented patient. *JAGS* 1986; **34**: 295–308.

13
Autonomic and Vegetative Functions

81. Urinary dysfunction secondary to Parkinson's disease is a diagnosis of exclusion

It is atypical for patients with mild Parkinson's disease to have prominent urinary dysfunction, and in this setting the presence of these symptoms should suggest an alternative diagnosis (see maxim 21). However, urinary dysfunction does occur in more severely affected patients (Murnaghan, 1961) and is not incompatible with the diagnosis of idiopathic parkinsonism.

Commonly, symptoms are of bladder irritability, and include urinary urgency, frequency and urge incontinence. These symptoms are confounded by the patient's motor problems, as the bradykinesia often prevents the patient from getting to the bathroom and disrobing in time to urinate. Obstructive symptoms, consisting of urinary hesitancy, urinary retention, slowing of urinary stream and post-void dribbling, also occur but are infrequent in idiopathic parkinsonism (Berger et al., 1987) and suggest another etiology. Some patients may have a mixed symptom pattern consisting of both urinary frequency and hesitancy.

Patients with levodopa-induced fluctuations may experience changes in urinary function that fluctuate with parkinsonism. Usually, urinary hesitancy or retention coincide with 'off' periods and improve with 'on' periods (Christmas et al., 1988), but some patients show the opposite pattern (Fitzmaurice et al., 1985).

Urodynamic studies in parkinsonian patients with urinary complaints reveal that 60–90% of the patients have detrusor hyperreflexia manifest by inappropriate bladder contractions at low bladder volumes (Berger et al., 1987; Khan et al., 1989; Pavlakis et al., 1983; Andersen and Bradley et al., 1976). This pattern is not unique to central neurologic disorders but may occasionally be seen with bladder neck obstruction. Rarely obstructive symptoms may occur due to detrusor areflexia or hyporeflexia, manifest by weak or absent bladder contraction.

Table 81.1 Patterns of urinary symptoms in patients with parkinsonism and urological compaints

Bladder dysfunction	Symptoms	Frequency
Irritative	Frequency, urgency	57–83%
Obstructive	Hesitancy, post-void dribbing	17–23%

Urethral sphincteric abnormalities have also been described in parkinsonism. Deficient voluntary control of the external urinary sphincter may predict urinary incontinence following prostatectomy (Staskin *et al.*, 1988; Andersen and Bradley, 1976). Denervation of the external urinary sphincter detected by sphincter electromyography is not a feature of idiopathic parkinsonism and strongly suggests the diagnosis of multiple system atrophy (Quinn *et al.*, 1989). Incoordination between detrusor contractions and relaxation of the internal and external urinary sphincter, termed detrusor–sphincter dyssynergia, is not common in parkinsonism and does not appear to cause obstruction (Andersen and Bradley, 1976; Berger *et al.*, 1987).

Urinary symptoms, particularly incontinence, should not be attributed to parkinsonism without excluding other causes for urinary dysfunction (Table 81.2). Historical features may aid in diagnosis; dysuria or an abrupt onset of urinary symptoms suggest coexistent urinary tract infection, and a change in urinary function that coincides with changes in medications may suggest drug-induced dysfunction. Physical examination should include evaluation of perineal sensation, the rectum for masses and fecal impaction, and anal sphincter tone and voluntary and reflex contraction. Bedside urological evaluation should include measurement of post-void residual volume, which should be less than 100 ml; larger volumes are an indication for further evaluation by a urologist familiar with neurologic abnormalities of the bladder. 'In and out' catheterization should be followed by one or two doses of co-trimoxazole to prevent a bladder infection; patients with known cardiac valvular abnormalities should receive a short course of antibacterial prophylaxis.

Treatment, of course, depends upon diagnosis. Recognition of drug-induced urinary dysfunction is important because it is common and readily treated. Anticholinergics, in particular, are a very common offender. They may produce obstructive symptoms, or they may cause partial urinary retention leading to urinary frequency and urgency. Though less common, similar side-effects may occur with Sinemet, dopamine agonists, sedative/hypnotics, and a large number of other drugs. For urinary frequency and urgency, peripherally acting anticholinergics may blunt detrusor contractions and reduce symptoms. Effective drugs include oxybutynin, usually administered at 5 mg, 1–4 times per day, and propantheline, 7.5–15 mg, 2–4 times per day.

Table 81.2 Etiology of urinary incontinence in the elderly

Transient and new-onset incontinence	Urinary tract infection
	Medications
	Fecal impaction
Chronic incontinence	Parkinsonism
	Lack of mobility
	Anatomic stress incontinence (women)
	Bladder-neck obstruction (prostate in men)
	Other peripheral or central neurological disorders
	Dementia or apathy

Treatment of obstructive symptoms is more difficult. In patients with increased symptoms during 'off' periods, a voiding schedule should be designed to coincide with periods of improved motor function. Patients with anatomical obstruction from prostatic hypertrophy should be considered for surgery only if obstruction can be demonstrated with urodynamic studies. Special care should be taken when considering surgery in these patients as there is a relatively high risk of post-surgical incontinence. Patients with poor voluntary sphincter control are at especially high risk (Staskin et al., 1987). Likewise, women with complaints of stress incontinence must be carefully evaluated with urodynamic studies before recommending surgery (Kahn et al., 1989). Patients with nonobstructive, overflow incontinence may require intermittent self-catheterization to avoid the complications of urosepsis or renal insufficiency resulting from hydronephrosis.

Nondrug treatment may include providing bedside commodes and scheduled voiding programs in patients with significant immobility due to parkinsonism. For management of incontinence, options include an external collection device, incontinence pads, or indwelling catheters. Finally, 'incontinence clinics' and lay organizations for the incontinent (see the appendix) may provide useful information in managing incontinence (Wells and Diokno, 1989).

82.   Sexual dysfunction is a common and multifactorial problem in Parkinson's disease.

Sexual dysfunction is a very common cause of dissatisfaction in patients with parkinsonism. In one series, two-thirds of patients, especially male patients and their normal female partners, reported some problem with sexual functioning (Brown et al., 1990). Although prevalent, sexual dysfunction may or may not be more frequent in idiopathic parkinsonism than in other chronic disorders; men with arthritis, for example, also have a high prevalence of sexual dysfunction (Lipe *et al.*, 1990). Because sexual difficulties are such a common cause of distress, healthcare providers should offer the patient an opportunity to discuss these concerns; questions regarding sexual functioning should be included in the review of systems and the provider should be prepared to initiate evaluation and management.

The most common sexual complaint is decreased sexual activity which may be due to alterations in autonomic, somatic or psychological function (Table 82.1). Less commonly hypersexuality or sexual delusions are a problem.

Erectile dysfunction or impotence is a particularly common complaint, reported by 60% of male patients (Brown *et al.*, 1990). It should be stressed, though, that there are numerous causes for impotence. Like other autonomic symptoms in patients with parkinsonism, impotence should not be attributed to parkinsonism without first conducting a thorough search for other, treatable conditions (Table 82.2). Although impotence can occur with idiopathic parkinsonism, it is atypical early in the course of the illness; if it does occur, particularly if coupled with severe constipation or urinary incontinence, the possibility of multiple system atrophy should be considered (maxim 25).

Adverse effects of antiparkinsonian medications are the most common cause of remediable sexual dysfunction. Tranquilizers, sedatives and beta-blocking agents are especially prone to cause impotence, but numerous other drugs may also cause erectile dysfunction. Anticholinergics or tricyclic antidepressants may cause mucosal dryness and consequently dyspareunia because of inadequate lubrication.

In addition to a review of medications, evaluation of sexual dysfunction should include a sexual and psychological history. Gradual, progressive decline in sexual function generally implicates an organic rather than psychological cause for the dysfunction. Examination should focus on perineal sensation, presence of an anal wink and autonomic functions. Laboratory screening should detect diabetes mellitus, hyperprolactinemia and

Table 82.1   Sexual dysfunction in parkinsonism

Autonomic symptoms	Decreased erectile ability
	Premature or delayed ejaculation
	Decreased mucosal lubrication
	Coexistent urinary and bowel dysfunction
Somatic symptoms	Difficulty in foreplay and satisfactory coital positioning, due to bradykinesia, dyskinesia, tremor, or dystonia
Psychological symptoms	Decreased arousal and interest by patient or sexual partner
	Sexual delusions
	Hypersexuality

Table 82.2   Common causes of impotence and other sexual dysfunction

Endocrinopathies	Hyperprolactinemia
	Hypogonadism
	Hypo- or hyperthyroidism
Spinal cord lesions	
Sensory neuropathies	Sacral root or cauda equina syndromes
	Sacral plexopathies
Autonomic neuropathies	Diabetes mellitus
	Renal insufficiency
	Alcoholism
	Other
Peripheral vascular diseases	
Urological disorders	Sequelae of abdominal prostatectomy
	Peyronies disease

Drugs and medications	*Antihypertensives*	*Psychotropic agents*
	Alpha-methyldopa	Neuroleptics (also associated
	Clonidine	with retrograde
	Diuretics	ejaculation)
	Beta-blockers	Lithium
	Reserpine	Tricyclic antidepressants
		Anticholinergics
		Sedatives
		Tetrabenazine
	Others	*Drugs of abuse*
	Cimetidine	Marijuana
	Estrogens	Cocaine
	Digoxin	Opiates
	Ethanol	
Psychogenic dysfunction	Depression	
	Anxiety	
	Sexual partner's attitude, libido, etc.	

Source: Modified from Seagrave *et al.* (1985)

hypogonadism. At this point it is necessary to assess the importance of the sexual relation to the couple and decide whether further workup and intervention is appropriate. For some couples the sexual relation is not of sufficient priority to warrant the trouble and expense. For other couples, urological or psychological referral is appropriate to continue the evaluation and initiate treatment.

Treatment of sexual dysfunction is multidisciplinary, and may involve neurologists, internists, urologists, vascular surgeons, and psychologists or psychiatrists. Treatment options include reducing or discontinuing drugs implicated in causing impotence, treatment of concomitant depression, psychological counselling and instructions in alternative physical interactions if intercourse is difficult or impossible. Adjusting antiparkinsonian therapy to increase mobility and decrease involuntary movements and timing love-making during optimal motor function will improve sexual function. Treatment aimed specifically at organic impotence includes intracavernosal injection of drugs, vascular surgery, and vacuum constriction devices. Finally, implantation of a penile prosthesis is a viable option in some patients, and parkinsonism should not be viewed as a contraindication for this treatment (Krane *et al.*, 1989).

Hypersexuality is a rare but well publicized side-effect of antiparkinsonian medications, including levodopa, selegiline, and dopamine agonists (Uitti *et al.*, 1989). It is more common in men. Hypersexuality may occur as an ongoing preoccupation in patients with otherwise clear sensoriums, or may accompany hypomania or delirium. Hypersexuality may coexist with impotence in males. The hypersexuality may be dose-dependent, and may limit the amount of levodopa that may be taken (Quinn *et al.*, 1983). Reduction or withdrawal of the dopaminergic agents stops the hypersexual behavior if behavioral modification is ineffective.

A final type of sexual problem is sexual delusions and hallucinations. Most frequently the patient imagines that the spouse is covertly having an affair or constantly masturbating. Some patients have hallucinations in which their spouse is involved in sexual activities with people and animals. These delusions and hallucinations may occur in a patient who is otherwise reasonably cogent; they may be very disturbing to both patient and spouse. Lowering the levodopa will give relief, but often at the expense of unacceptable increase in parkinsonism. Because the hallucinations and delusions are particularly prevalent at night, enhancing sleep is beneficial for some patients.

83. *Orthostatic hypotension is commonly caused by drugs and less commonly caused by disease*

An orthostatic drop in blood pressure occurs in many patients with parkinsonism. Symptoms vary; some patients report few or no symptoms, despite standing systolic blood pressures as low as 70 mmHg, while others experience dizziness, lightheadedness, weakness, blurred vision, syncope, or falls. Orthostatic hypotension, which appears to be asymptomatic, remains a risk factor for falls and syncope (Lipsitz, 1989).

Orthostatic hypotension is detected by measuring the blood pressure (1) after the patient has been supine for 5 minutes, (2) immediately upon standing (or sitting with feet dangling), and (3) after standing for 2 minutes. Immediately on standing, the normal physiologic response is for the systolic blood pressure to fall, the diastolic blood pressure to remain the same or even rise slightly and the heart rate to accelerate, a response to decreased venous return to the heart due to pooling of blood in the lower extremity veins (Thomas *et al.*, 1981). An excessive fall of the systolic blood pressure and acceleration of heart rate may cause transient symptoms, termed 'poor postural adjustment'. A drop of 30 mmHg in systolic blood pressure and 15 mmHg in diastolic blood pressure provoked by assumption of the upright position or exercise, with symptoms, is one criterion for the diagnosis of orthostatic hypotension (Thomas *et al.*, 1981). There are two caveats in evaluating orthostatic blood pressure changes. First, in the elderly, cardio-acceleration (an increase of 10 or more beats per minute), a normal response to orthostatic hypotension caused by volume depletion, may be absent. Secondly, orthostatic hypotension may vary markedly during the day, partially in relation to meals and medication ingestion; the absence of an orthostatic drop on one measurement does not exclude large drops at other times during the day.

Postural hypotension has many causes and may be a multifactorial problem in the elderly (Table 83.1). The most common cause, which is also treatable, is drug-induced hypotension. Hypotension is a common side-effect of levodopa and dopamine agonists, and is especially prominent in the newly treated patient and in the elderly. It may be lessened by initially administering low doses of dopamine agonists at bedtime, and then slowly titrating the dose upward. However, hypotension may limit the dose or the frequency of treatment with levodopa or dopamine agonists. It may occur completely independently of any beneficial motor effect of antiparkinsonian drugs. It need not be an early side-effect and may emerge over time in patients who previously did not experience hypotension. Orthostatic hypotension may fluctuate in severity throughout the day along with motor or sensory symptoms in patients on chronic levodopa therapy (see maxim 52). When 'on' the patient has orthostatic hypotension and when 'off' may even be hypertensive.

Antihypertensives and nitrates are other classes of drugs which commonly produce orthostatic changes, but almost every centrally active drug has the ability to produce hypotension (Table 83.1).

Postural hypotension can accompany otherwise typical parkinsonism. Such patients have a loss of the preganglionic cell bodies in the intermediolateral column of the spinal cord as well as Lewy body inclusions in autonomic ganglia. However, physicians should remember that prominent, severe orthostatic hypotension is unusual in mildly affected patients and that multiple system atrophy should be suspected in such circumstances (see maxim 25).

Orthostatic hypotension may also result from a variety of other neurological or systemic illnesses, including autonomic neuropathies, intercurrent infections, dehydration or salt deprivation, and prolonged immobility (Table 83.1).

Treatment of orthostatic hypotension should be tailored to symptoms, rather than signs. Asymptomatic hypotension, even if marked, may not require treatment (recalling, however, that it may be a risk factor for falls). Symptomatic treatment includes reduction or elimination of antiparkinsonian drugs and other medications, as the medical condition permits. Usually, drug-induced hypotension lessens or resolves quickly following elimination of the offending medication. However, selegiline is an exception; it may accentuate levodopa-induced hypotension, and this effect may persist for weeks after discontinuing the drug. Levodopa-induced hypotension generally occurs transiently after taking a dose. This peak-dose hypotension may be treated by reducing the dose of levodopa or by slowing the absorption of the drug by either taking it with small meals or using controlled-release preparations.

If modification of the drug regimen does not reduce symptomatic hypotension or if orthostatic hypotension occurs in the absence of drug therapy, fludrocortisone, a potent mineralocorticoid, may be helpful. At low doses (0.1 mg/day) it enhances the response to norepinephrine and improves standing blood pressure. At higher doses (0.2–1.0 mg/day) it increases blood pressure by promoting retention of sodium, thus expanding extracellular volume by retention of sodium. Its use requires a liberal intake of salt. As a consequence of sodium retention and volume expansion, fludrocortisone may cause edema of the lower extremities or may even trigger or worsen congestive heart failure. Fludrocortisone promotes excretion of potassium. Thus, serum electrolytes should be periodically monitored to avoid hypokalemia. Fludrocortisone commonly produces supine systolic and diastolic hypertension; the risks of the recumbent hypertension must be balanced against that of the standing hypotension.

Table 83.1   Causes of orthostatic hypotension

Parkinsonian syndromes	Idiopathic parkinsonism with central autonomic involvement
	Multiple system atrophy
Drugs	Levodopa
	Dopamine agonists
	Amantadine
	Selegiline (especially combined with levodopa)
	Antidepressants
	Sedative hypnotics
	Antipsychotics
	Benzodiazepines
	Analgesics
	Antihypertensives
	Vasodilators
	Diuretics
Coexistent diseases	Autonomic neuropathies (diabetes, alcohol)
	Brainstem and spinal cord lesions
	Dehydration, intercurrent illness
	Decreased oral intake from dysphagia
	Decreased salt intake
	Immobility

Other drugs employed in the treatment of orthostatic hypotension are less consistently effective, but may be beneficial in individual patients with recalcitrant hypotension. These include sympathomimetics (ephedrine, Ritalin), beta-blockers, alpha-2 antagonists, dihydroergotamine (a venoconstrictor), indomethacin or other nonsteroidal anti-inflammatory medications, vasopressin and large doses of salt tablets (reviewed in Thomas *et al.*, 1981). Domperidone, a peripherally active dopamine antagonist, has a slight hypertensive effect by itself and may partially block levodopa or dopamine agonist-induced hypotension.

Nonpharmacological management may be sufficient alone or may be combined with pharmacologic management. One simple treatment is to liberalize salt and fluid intake. Elevation of the head of the bed by 5–20 degrees induces a mild hypotensive stress when recumbent, thereby promoting renin release and retention of water and sodium; standing blood pressure may consequently be improved. Pressure stockings, panty hose or even antigravity suits are helpful, but are cumbersome to apply; use by elderly, frail parkinsonian patients may be difficult.

Elimination of other environmental causes of peripheral vasodilation may be helpful. Hot baths may be contraindicated. Hot, humid weather promotes faintness, to the degree that some patients are unable to venture outside of air-conditioned buildings in the summer. Alcohol induces syncopal symptoms by producing peripheral vasodilation, and should be avoided in patients with severe hypotension. Parkinsonian patients may be particularly prone to postprandial hypotension; large meals are best avoided and a period of rest scheduled after each meal. The patient and

Table 83.2   Treatment of orthostatic hypotension

A. Elimination or reduction of hypotensive medications
B. Pharmacological management
    Fludrocortisone
    Propranolol
    Clonidine
    Yohimbine
    Ephedrine
    Caffeine
    Indomethacin
    Domperidone
C. Non-pharmacological management
    Sodium chloride tablets
    Elevation of the head of the bed 5–20 degrees
    Changing position slowly
    Pressure stockings, pantyhose
    Liberalizing salt and fluid intake
    Avoidance of hot weather, hot tubs or baths, alcohol, large meals
    Patient and caregiver education

caregiver should be educated about hypotensive symptoms, the need both to change position slowly, and to sit or lie down when orthostatic symptoms appear.

84.   *Excessive sweating is embarrassing*

Gowers (1888) and Charcot (1877) first described excessive sweating, sometimes confined to the most affected limb, in patients with parkinsonism. Patients may complain of excessive sweating and, in a few patients, paroxysms of profuse sweating necessitate changes of clothing or bed sheets; these symptoms are a very embarrassing and discomforting aspect of parkinsonism. Qualitative and quantitative studies of sweating in parkinsonism have demonstrated that patients exposed to heat tend to sweat more in the upper body, particularly the neck and head, than do controls (Appenzeller and Goss, 1971; Goetz *et al.*, 1986; Turkka and Myllyla, 1987). Sweating is variably reported as decreased over the trunk and lower extremities (Appenzeller and Goss, 1971; Goetz *et al.*, 1986, Turkka and Myllyla, 1987). An asymmetry in sweating, correlating with an asymmetry in the severity of the parkinsonism, has not been described in recent studies – in contradistinction to the clinical observations of Gowers and Charcot.

Treatment of troublesome sweating is problematic. Anticholinergics might be expected to ameliorate excessive sweating because the autonomic innervation of the sweat glands is by cholinergic postganglionic sympathetic fibers. However, anticholinergics are generally an ineffective treatment for this problem. Propranolol has been reported to decrease paroxysms of sweating (Tanner *et al.*, 1982) although in our experience the beta-adrenergic antagonists have not been effective. Often the excessive sweating is most apparent when the patient is 'off'; levodopa reduces or abolishes the abnormalities of sweating (Goetz *et al.*, 1986). Understandably then, reduction of the fluctuating response with dopamine agonists will reduce excess sweating (Tanner, 1987).

Decreased sweating may occur in multiple system atrophies but is rarely a source of complaints.

85.   *Dyspnea is a rare but disabling side-effect of levodopa*

A variety of respiratory abnormalities have been documented in parkinsonism (see Table 85.1) and have been attributed to both motor abnormalities of respiratory, laryngeal and pharyngeal muscles as part of the parkinsonian motor dysfunction (Nakano *et al.*, 1972; Vincken *et al.*, 1978) as well as

Table 85.1   Respiratory abnormalities of parkinsonism

Restrictive	Decreased maximum ventilatory volume, decreased maximum expiratory flow rate (FEV1) attributed to rigidity of chest wall, poor posture, and inability to perform coordinated, rhythmical movements for respiratory testing
Obstructive	Involuntary movements of the glottis and supraglottic structures. Vocal cord paresis, particularly in multiple system atrophy
Tachypnea, irregular respiration, dyspnea	Occurring with levodopa-induced dyskinesia of respiratory muscles
	Occurring with levodopa treatment but without dyskinesia and presumably of central origin
	Occurring during 'off' periods and perhaps related to anxiety as an 'off' phenomenon
Sighs, gasps	Occurring in postencephalitic parkinsonism and in multiple system atrophies

to abnormalities of pontomedullary respiratory centers and their supranuclear connections. Dopaminergic interneurons are found within the peripheral chemoreceptors located in the carotid and aortic bodies (Berger et al., 1977) and dopaminergic nerve terminals in the vicinity of brainstem respiratory centers (Mueller et al., 1982). Hence dopaminergic agents might directly influence respiration by affecting on the peripheral chemoreceptors for central respiratory centers and indirectly influence respiration by altering respiratory and airway musculature via effects on the basal ganglia.

The respiratory complaint most commonly encountered in parkinsonian patients is dyspnea, occurring almost exclusively in levodopa-treated patients, and most commonly related to administration of levodopa or dopaminergic agonists. Affected patients have rapid and irregular respirations accompanied by dyspnea 15–60 minutes after drug ingestion which persists for minutes to hours. For some patients the dyspnea is associated with chorea of abdominal and respiratory muscles suggesting that the dyspnea may be secondary to the dyskinesia (Weiner et al., 1978). In other patients, however, dyspnea may occur without chorea in the respiratory muscles and may be attributed to a central effect on respiratory centers (Zupnick et al., 1990). In both groups of patients, blood gases are consistent with hyperventilation during the episodes; oxygenation is more than adequate. The dyspnea is very uncomfortable for the patient and generally requires reducing, substituting or completely withdrawing dopaminergic drugs. Dopamine antagonists will block the dyspnea but will likely worsen the parkinsonism.

Dyspnea associated with rapid shallow respiration may also occur during 'off' periods in patients with a fluctuating response to levodopa; this dyspnea may be related to a re-emergence of parkinsonism and the restrictive and obstructive respiratory abnormalities (Ilson *et al.*, 1983). However, some patients develop marked anxiety and depression during 'off' periods, causing or contributing to the dyspnea. Dopamine agonists and antidepressants may reduce the dyspnea in this situation.

Exertional dyspnea has been noted in untreated parkinsonian patients and attributed to restrictive disease (Nugent *et al.*, 1958). This complaint, however, is uncommon in our experience. When restrictive disease becomes clinically apparent, these patients generally have such disability that they do not exercise enough to experience exertional dyspnea.

Respiratory failure secondary to vocal cord paresis is relatively common in patients with multiple system atrophy (Williams *et al.*, 1979). Because of the concomitant restrictive pulmonary dysfunction in these patients, they rarely develop stridor. Extremely loud snoring at night is the usual tip-off to cord paresis. Sleep apnea and respiratory failure may eventually develop, requiring tracheostomy.

Sighs and gasps interspersed in an otherwise normal respiratory pattern are observed in patients with parkinsonism. Sighs and gasps were particularly common in patients with postencephalitic parkinsonism; now these symptoms often indicate that the patient has multiple system atrophy.

86.   *Symptomatic cardiac arrhythmias are an uncommon adverse effect of dopaminergic drugs*

Dopaminergic drugs can potentially affect cardiac rhythm via peripheral or central mechanisms but peripheral mechanisms appear to be pre-eminent. Dopaminergically induced arrhythmias are mediated through the beta-adrenergic receptor both by direct activation of the receptor, and by enhancement of norepinephrine release from sympathetic nerve terminals (Hoffman and Lefkowitz, 1990).

When levodopa was introduced, adverse effects which caused much concern included cardiac arrhythmias, especially as early reports indicated increased atrial and ventricular ectopic contractions (Goldberg and Whitsett, 1971). In practice, however, few serious cardiac arrhythmias were documented (Hunter *et al.*, 1971; Jenkins *et al.*, 1972). The combination of aromatic amino acid decarboxylase inhibitors with levodopa decreased peripheral production of dopamine and reduced ectopic activity (Mars and Krall, 1971). Despite these reassuring reports, some patients undoubtedly have increased ectopic contractions, including trigeminy, when plasma levodopa levels are increased – even in the presence of decarboxylase inhibitors. The clinical significance of this ectopy is unclear; it is usually asymptomatic and is generally not treated. Nevertheless, if dopaminergic

agents can be decreased without significant loss of antiparkinsonian efficacy, dose reduction would seem a prudent course to pursue in affected
patients. If treatment of the ectopy is required, a beta-adrenergic antagonist
such as propranolol is a logical choice since the arrhythmic effects of levodopa are mediated by the beta-adrenergic receptor (Goldberg and Whitsett,
1971). The peripheral dopamine antagonist, domperidone, may also reduce
cardiac premature contractions caused by dopaminergic drugs (Quinn *et
al.*, 1985).

The dopamine agonist, pergolide, was also initially thought to cause
cardiac arrhythmias (Leibowitz *et al.*, 1981). However, subsequent studies
failed to confirm any cardiotoxicity of the drug (Tanner *et al.*, 1985); the
current clinical impression is that cardiac effects are no more common with
pergolide treatment than might usually be expected in this age group.

The final concern – cardiac arrhythmias resulting from an interaction
between anesthetic agents and dopaminergic drugs (Goldberg and Whitsett, 1971) – also has not materialized as a significant problem (see maxim
95).

87.   Chronic constipation is common

Constipation, defined as less than three bowel movements per week, is
commonly encountered in the elderly and is even more prevalent in those
with parkinsonism. Within the long list of etiologies for chronic constipation (Tremaine, 1990), certain factors listed in Table 87.1 particularly
predispose the parkinsonian patient to constipation.

Table 87.1   Causes of constipation in parkinsonism

Dietary	Inadequate dietary fiber intake
	Inadequate fluid intake
Activity	Physical inactivity
	Poor bowel habits
Impaired defecation	Pelvic floor dysfunction
	Inadequate abdominal and diaphragmatic contractions
Autonomic dysfunction	Idiopathic Parkinson's disease
	Multiple system atrophy (Shy–Drager syndrome)
	Depression
Drugs	Anticholinergics (antiparkinsonian agents, antidepressants)
	Iron
	Nonsteroidal anti-inflammatory agents
	Opiate analgesics
	Sympathomimetics (ephedrine, etc)

Constipation is generally related to decreased colonic transit time, reflecting inadequate colonic propulsive motility. However, recently attention has been directed to anismus, a dyssynergy of pelvic floor muscle contractions which prevents rectal emptying in some parkinsonian patients with constipation (Mathers et al., 1989). In these patients attempts to defecate produce contraction rather than relaxation of the striated anal sphincter; defecation is obstructed. This dysfunctional defecation is improved by dopaminergic drugs in most patients. The prevalence of anismus in constipated parkinsonian patients is not known, nor is there sufficient experience to suggest when to suspect this problem or ways to treat it. Botulinum toxin injections into the anal sphincter have been suggested as a possible treatment for this problem.

A stepwise approach to constipation is as follows:

1. Determine that the patient has constipation; that is, fewer than three bowel movements per week. The abdominal radiograph may be the best determinant of constipation; a large number of patients complain of constipation but have no objective evidence of retained stool by rectal exam or X-ray (Donald et al., 1985).

2. Rule out other colon and rectal disorders that could cause constipation; utilize the history, rectal exam and other tests if indicated. Consider current drugs that might be contributing to constipation and modify the drug regimen if possible.

3. Improve bowel habits. Encourage the patient to try to have a bowel movement at a regular time, taking advantage of times of naturally higher gut motility, after meals and exercise. Also this time should coincide with an 'on' time if the patient has a fluctuating response to levodopa. Make certain that the patient has a comfortable, private toilet. Increase physical exercise, even if the patient is only able to walk in the hall once or twice per day.

4. Increase stool bulk by increasing dietary fiber to 20–30 g/day – by increasing the intake of grains and cereals. Such dietary changes should be gradual to minimize bloating, flatulence and abdominal discomfort. Psyllium and methylcellulose can be used as bulking agents if augmentation of dietary fiber is not possible or tolerated. A critical aspect of these strategies to increase stool bulk is adequate hydration; without 1.5–2 liters of fluid per day, the bulk-forming agents may exacerbate rather than improve the constipation.

5. Stool softeners (docusate salts) and lubricants (mineral oil) have a less clearly defined role in treating constipation (Castle, 1989) but may be helpful for some patients. Mineral oil should not be used as a lubricant in any patient with difficulty swallowing because it is toxic to the lungs if aspirated. In addition, mineral oil can interfere with the absorption of fat-soluble vitamins, cause a foreign body reaction in the intestinal mucosa and can leak through the anal sphincter. For all these reasons, mineral oil is rarely indicated. Stool softeners and lubricants are unlikely to relieve constipation if other measures are not instituted as well.

6. The osmotic laxative, lactulose, can be employed if the steps above are not effective. Lactulose, a nonabsorbable sugar, works by increasing the water content of the stool; 15–30 ml once or twice per day may be used chronically. Gas, bloating and cramping are side-effects that may limit the use of lactulose.

The other orally administered osmotic laxatives are magnesium (Milk of Magnesia) and phosphate salts which are effective on an 'as needed' basis. The chronic use of magnesium and phosphate salts can lead to fluid and electrolyte disturbances and is discouraged.

7. Glycerin suppositories stimulate defecation by causing retention of fluid in the rectum; they are more effective if given before periods of increased gut motility. Many other suppositories contain irritative laxatives and, as discussed below, should be used cautiously. Tapwater enemas are safe but frequent use may reduce anal sphincter tone and lead to rectal incontinence.

8. Irritative laxatives – those containing senna, cascara, bisacodyl and phenophthalein – should be used sparingly to avoid damage to the colonic smooth muscle and intrinsic nerves which can lead to the dilated, atonic 'cathartic colon'. However, this complication usually results from taking large doses of irritant laxatives for 20–40 years and should not be a reason to avoid these agents altogether. The irritant laxatives should be used, when all the steps above are unsuccessful, on a less than once per week basis.

Fecal impaction is a complication of constipation. Impaction may present with anorexia, nausea, abdominal discomfort and distension, diarrhea, fecal incontinence and confusion. Most impactions are in the rectum and palpable by rectal exam. Impaction may be elsewhere in the colon and require abdominal X-ray for diagnosis. Stool consistency may vary from soft to hard. Disimpaction usually requires manual fragmentation of the fecal mass. If above the reach of the fingers, lavage guided by sigmoidos-

Table 87.2   Common anticonstipation agents

Generic	Example	Dose
Bulk agents		
Bran	–	10–20 g/day
Psyllium	Metamucil	Up to 30 g/day
Methylcellulose	Citrucel	Up to 6 g/day
Stool softener		
Docusate sodium	Colase	100–500 mg/day
Osmotic		
Lactulose	Chronulac	15–60 ml/day
Sorbitol	–	15–60 ml/day
Magnesium hydroxide	Milk of Magnesia	15–60 ml/day
Sodium phosphate	Fleet enema	
Glycerin	–	Suppository
Stimulant		
Bisacodyl	Dulcolax	5 mg tab, 10 mg suppository
Phenolphthalein	Modane	30–200 mg/day
Anthraquinone	Senokot	1–4 tsp/day

Source: Adapted from Castle (1989) and Brunton (1990)

copy may be necessary. Fragmentation of the impacted stool is followed by stimulant suppositories and sodium phosphate or tapwater enemas (Wrenn, 1989).

References

Andersen JT, Bradley WE. Cystometric, sphincter, and electromyelographic abnormalities in Parkinson's disease. *J Urol* 1975; **116**: 75–8.

Appenzeller O, Goss JE. Autonomic deficits in Parkinson's syndrome. *Arch Neurol* 1971; **24**: 50–87.

Berger AJ, Mitchell RA, Severinghaus JW. Regulation of respiration. *N Engl J Med* 1977; **297**: 92–7, 138–43, 194–201.

Berger Y, Blaivas JG, DeLaRocha ER, Salinas JM. Urodynamic findings in Parkinson's disease. *J Urol* 1987; **138**: 836–8.

Brown RG, Jahanshahi M, Quinn N, Marsden CD. Sexual function in patients with Parkinson's disease and their partners. *J Neurol Neurosurg Psychiatry* 1990; **53**: 480–6.

Brunton LL. Agents affecting gastrointestinal water flux and motility, digestants and bile acids. In: Gilman AG, Rall TW, Nies AS, Taylor P (eds), *The Pharmacological Basis of Therapeutics*, 8th edn. New York: Pergamon Press, 1990: 914–21.

Castle SC. Constipation: endemic in the elderly? *Med Clin NA* 1989; **73**: 1497–509.

Charcot JM. *Lectures on the Diseases of the Nervous System* (Trans Sigerson G). London: The New Sydenham Society, 1877.

Christmas TJ, Chapple CR, Lees AJ, *et al.* Role of subcutaneous apomorphine in parkinsonian voiding dysfunction. *Lancet* 1988; **2**: 1451–3.

Cosio MG. Involvement of upper-airway muscles in extrapyramidal disorders. *N Engl J Med* 1984; **311**: 438–42.

Donald IP, Smith RG, Cruikshank JG, Elton RA, Stoddart ME. A study of constipation in the elderly living at home. *Gerontology* 1985; **31**: 112–18.

Fitzmaurice H, Fowler CJ, Rickards D. *et al.* Micturition disturbance in Parkinson's disease. *Br J Urol* 1985; **57**: 652–6.

Goetz CG, Lutge W, Tanner CM. Autonomic dysfunction in Parkinson's disease. *Neurology* 1986; **36**: 73–5

Goldberg LI, Whitsett TL. Cardiovascular effects of levodopa. *Clin Pharmacol Ther* 1971; **12**: 376–82.

Gowers WR. *Diseases of the Nervous System*. Philadelphia: F. Blakiston, Son & Co., 1888.

Hoffman BB, Lefkowitz RJ. Catecholamines and sympathomimetic drugs. In: Gilman AG, Rall TW, Nies AS, Taylor P (eds), *The Pharmacological Basis of Therapeutics*, 8th edn. New York: Pergamon Press, 1990: 187–243.

Hunter KR, Hollman A, Laurence DR, Stern GM. Levodopa in parkinsonian patients with heart-disease. *Lancet* 1971; **1**: 932–4.

Ilson J, Braun N, Fahn S. Respiratory fluctuations in Parkinson's disease. *Neurology* 1983; **33** (suppl 2): 113.

Jenkins RB, Mendelson SH, Lamid S, Klawans HL. Levodopa therapy of patients with parkinsonism and heart disease. *Br Med J* 1972; **3**: 512–14.

Khan Z, Starer P, Bhola A. Urinary incontinence in female Parkinson's disease patients: pitfalls of diagnosis. *Urology* 1989; **33**: 486–9.

Krane RJ, Goldstein I, Saenz de Tehada I. Impotence. *N Engl J Med* 1989; **321**: 1648–59.

Leibowitz M, Lieberman A, Goldstein M, *et al.* The cardiac effects of pergolide, a potent and long-acting dopamine agonist. *Clin Pharm Ther* 1981; **30**: 718–23.

Lipe H, Longstreth WT, Burd TD, Linde M. Sexual function in married men with

Parkinson's disease compared to married men with arthritis. *Neurology* 1990; **40**: 1347–49.

Lipsitz LA. Orthostatic hypotension in the elderly. *N Engl J Med* 1989; **321**: 952–7.

Mars H, Krall J. L-DOPA and cardiac arrhythmias. *N Engl J Med* 1971; **285**: 1437.

Mathers SE, Kempster PA, Law PJ, *et al.* Anal sphincter dysfunction in Parkinson's disease. *Arch Neurol* 1989; **46**: 1061–4.

Mueller RA, Lundberg DBA, Breese GR, Hedner J, Hedner T, Jonason J. The neuropharmacology of respiratory control. *Pharmacol Rev* 1982; **34**: 255–85.

Murnaghan GF. Neurogenic disorders of the bladder in parkinsonism. *Br J Urol* 1961; **3**: 403–9.

Nakano KK, Bass H, Tyler HR. Levodopa in Parkinson's disease: effect on pulmonary function. *Arch Intern Med* 1972; **130**: 346–8.

Nugent CA, Harris HW, Cohn J, Smith CC, Tyler FH. Dyspnea as a symptom in Parkinson's disease. *Am Rev Tuber* 1958; **78**: 682–91.

Pavlakis AJ, Siroky MB, Goldstein I, Krane RJ. Neurourologic findings in Parkinson's disease. *J Urol* 1983; **129**: 80–3.

Quinn NP, Eardley I, Fowler CJ, Kirby RS, Marsden CD, Bannister R. The role of urethral sphincter electromyography in the differential diagnosis of parkinsonism. *Neurology* 1989; **39** (suppl 1): 142.

Quinn N, Parkes D, Jackson G, Upward J. Cardiotoxicity of domperidone. *Lancet* 1985; **2**: 724.

Quinn N, Toone B, Lang AE, Marsden CD, Parkes JD. Dopa dose-dependent sexual deviation. *Br J Psychiat* 1983; **142**: 296–8.

Seagraves RT, Schoenberg HW. *Diagnosis and Treatment of Erectile Disturbance: A Guide for Clinicians.* New York: Plenum, 1985.

Staskin DS, Vardi Y, Siroky MB. Post-prostatectomy continence in the parkinsonian patient: the significance of poor voluntary sphincter control. *J Urol* 1988; **140**: 117–18.

Tanner CM, Goetz CG, Glantz RH, Glatt SL, Klawans HL. Pergolide mesylate and idiopathic Parkinson's disease. *Neurology* 1982; **32**: 1175–79.

Tanner CM, Goetz CG, Klawans HL. Paroxysmal drenching sweats in idiopathic parkinsonism: response to propranolol. *Neurology* 1982; **32** (suppl 2): 162.

Tanner CM, Chablani R, Goetz CG, Klawans HL. Pergolide mesylate: lack of cardiac toxicity in patients with cardiac disease. *Neurology* 1985; **35**: 918–21.

Thomas JE, Schirger A, Fealey RD, Sheps SG. Ortnostatic hypotension, *Mayo clinic Proc* 1981; **56**: 117–25.

Tremaine WJ. Chronic constipation: causes and management. *Hosp Pract* 1990; (4): 89–100.

Turkka JT, Myllyla VV. Sweating dysfunction in Parkinson's disease. *Eur Neurol* 1987; **26**: 1–7.

Uitti RJ, Tanner CM, Rajput AH, Goetz CG, Klawans HL, Thiessen B. Hypersexuality with antiparkinsonian therapy. *Clin Neuropharmacol* 1989; **12**: 375–83.

Vincken WG, Gauthier SG, Dollfuss RE, Hanson RE, Darauay CM, Weiner WJ, Goetz CG, Nausieda PA, Klawans HL. Respiratory dyskinesias: extrapyramidal dysfunction and dyspnea. *Ann Intern Med* 1978; **88**: 327–31.

Weiner WJ, Goetz CG, Nausieda PA, Klawans HL. Respiratory dyskinesias: extrapyramidal dysfunction and dyspnea. *Ann Int Med*; **88**: 327–31.

Wells TJ, Diokno AC. Urinary incontinence in the elderly. *Seminars in Neurol* 1989; **9**: 60–7.

Williams AC, Hanson D, Calne DB. Vocal cord paralysis in the Shy–Drager syndrome. *J Neurol Neurosurg Psychiat* 1979; **42**: 151–3.

Wrenn K. Fecal impaction. *New Engl J Med* 1989; **321**: 658–62.

Zupnick HM, Brown LK, Miller A, Moros DA. Respiratory dysfunction due to L-dopa therapy for parkinsonism: diagnosis using serial pulmonary function tests and respiratory inductive plethysmography. *Am J Med* 1990; **89**: 109–14.

14
Special Considerations

88. *There are a variety of ways to cope with speech and communication problems*

In the later stages of parkinsonism the hypophonia and hypokinetic dysarthria can impose severe restrictions on effective communication, requiring patience and constant encouragement by the family. The soft mumbling speech is caused by poor control of respiration as well as bradykinesia and rigidity of the speech musculature. Long latencies and silences are punctuated by brief rushes of poorly articulated propulsive speech – as if the patient is trying to say everything in one short breath (also see maxim 12).

Levodopa therapy may improve speech by improving articulation and by shortening the latency between initiation of labial movement and speech. However, drug-induced respiratory and orobuccolingual dyskinesias, particularly dystonia, can produce a peak-dose deterioration of speech; thus, there may be a paradoxical improvement in speech and communication when the patient is 'off'. Commonly encountered dyskinesias that interfere with speech include: irregular panting respirations, tachypnea with dyspnea, protrusion or rolling of the tongue, lip smacking, and grimacing or chewing. Occasionally, patients may have laryngeal stridor or compulsive humming or whistling (Critchley, 1981).

Speech therapy consists of exercises designed for increasing breath support, increasing voice loudness and variation, improving articulation, and decreasing the rate of speech and the number of words with each breath. The best results from speech therapy are obtained early in the disease, when the spouse is involved and can remind and encourage the patient to use the techniques and practice the exercises daily. A marked improvement in speech may occur during the period of therapy, but the long-term benefits are harder to document (Yorkston *et al.*, 1988). Nevertheless, speech therapy is generally worthwhile when dysarthria first becomes symptomatic.

A variety of communication aids may be helpful. A voice amplifier can be useful if the main problem is hypophonia or the spouse is hard of hearing. A simple test to judge whether amplification will help is to take a length of tubing and have the patient talk into one end and the spouse listen at the other. If impaired articulation and/or uneven rate of speech are present, amplification may not help. Other types of augmentative communication aids may be necessary for patients with severe dysarthria and hypophonia. These range from simple alphabet or word charts to more sophisticated electronic devices with display, print, or speech synthesis options (Yorkston *et al.*, 1988). The catch is that by the time speech is so severely impaired as to require augmentative communication devices, manual dexterity is frequently too poor to operate the equipment effectively.

89. *Swallowing difficulties are common*

Patients at all stages of parkinsonism may have abnormalities of swallowing as demonstrated by modified barium swallow with video fluoroscopy. The most frequent abnormalities are delayed swallowing reflex, decreased pharyngeal peristalsis, decreased laryngeal elevation, and decreased tongue mobility (Bushmann *et al.*, 1989). The type and degree of abnormality cannot be predicted from the specific swallowing symptoms or from lack of complaints of dysphagia; asymptomatic patients can have significant abnormalities, including silent aspiration. Although a higher frequency of abnormalities is seen in more severely affected patients, about 50% of stage 1 and 2 patients also have abnormal barium swallow studies.

A variety of complaints may be voiced by the patient or spouse, such as choking, holding food in the mouth, and sticking of food and pills in the pharynx. The decrease in reflex swallowing leads to pooling of saliva, which further interferes with speech and swallowing and results in socially embarrassing drooling.

Choking is frequently reported by the patient and family (Edwards *et al.*, 1991) and is a tip-off both to disordered swallowing and to an increased risk of aspiration. However, clinically significant aspiration can occur in the absence of any respiratory symptoms. Silent aspiration is 'silent' because the patient develops pneumonia. Some signs that should arouse suspicion and lead to consideration of a barium swallow are listed in Table 89.1.

Unfortunately, treatment with levodopa improves swallowing only in a minority of patients (Bushmann *et al.*, 1989). Levodopa-induced improvement of general parkinsonian symptoms does not necessarily correlate with improvement in swallowing. Anticholinergics may impair swallowing; although they are sometimes prescribed for drooling, the underlying defect in reflex swallowing may not be improved and the resultant thickening of secretions may worsen the dysphagia. Papaya extract from a health-food store may be tried to decrease saliva production. Silent aspiration can

Table 89.1   Signs of silent aspiration

Altered voice quality – gurgling or rattling
Watering of the eyes after a swallow
Feeling of fullness or food sticking in throat
Complaints about or refusal to eat a particular food texture
Unexplained intermittent temperature spikes

be reduced by teaching the patient to protect the airway by the 'supraglottic swallow', in which patients are instructed to hold their breath, tilt the chin to the chest, swallow, cough, then swallow again (Bushmann *et al.*, 1989).

Severe dysphagia can lead to undernutrition. Body weight is a good and convenient indicator of nutritional status, and should, therefore, be regularly monitored. Some weight loss is a common (but poorly understood) consequence of having idiopathic parkinsonism; a loss of 10% or more of body weight over a period of time as short as three months is an indication of either undernutrition or another disease process and requires careful evaluation.

A feeding tube is rarely necessary in idiopathic parkinsonism, but is sometimes required for adequate nutrition or to protect the airway in patients with 'parkinsonism-plus' syndromes. The percutaneous endoscopic gastrostomy (PEG) is a much simpler technique than the gastrostomy and has fewer complications. The placement of a PEG may change meals from prolonged struggles, with insufficient food and liquid intake, to a more enjoyable experience; some patients take by mouth only what is easy and pleasurable and the PEG provides nutrition and fluid. Improved nutrition and hydration with a PEG may give the patient better overall health and well-being.

90.   *Dystonia has many etiologies in parkinsonism*

Dystonia is common in patients with parkinsonism, affecting up to one-third of patients chronically treated with levodopa (Poewe *et al.*, 1988) In most patients, dystonia is a manifestation of levodopa-induced dyskinesias (see maxim 59). However, dystonia and parkinsonism occur together in patients not receiving levodopa. In this setting this symptom has other diagnostic and treatment implications.

Dystonia either preceding or appearing concurrently with otherwise typical parkinsonism has long been recognized (Purves-Stewart, 1898). The symptom has a predilection for the lower extremities and feet, typically involving some combination of (1) dorsiflexion of the great toe (striatal toe), (2) plantar flexion of the other toes, and (3) inversion of the ankle. Other segmental and focal dystonias may occur, including cranial dystonia, torticollis, writer's cramp, limb dystonia and hemidystonia. If the dystonia is unilateral, the parkinsonian features generally begin ipsilaterally or are worse on the dystonic side. Dystonia is a much more common presenting symptom in patients with young onset of parkinsonism. Although the dystonia may be an incidental sign at the time the parkinsonism is diagnosed, it often causes as much disability as the parkinsonism itself (Klawans and Paleologos, 1986, LeWitt et al., 1986; Poewe et al., 1988). Dystonia can be either action-induced (i.e. appearing only during voluntary movement) or static (present at rest as well as during movement); the latter sometimes leads to contractures, further impairing use of the limb (Kyriakides and Hewer, 1988; Quinn et al., 1988).

Dystonia, or at least abnormal postures, are seen in 'parkinsonism plus' syndromes. Antecollis has been associated with multiple system atrophy (Quinn, 1989), and retrocollis with progressive supranuclear palsy. Other dystonias have also been reported, some of these relatively unusual syndromes, but accompanied by only minimal pathologic verification of the diagnosis (Rivest, 1990).

The coexistence of dystonia and parkinsonism may occur in a variety of neurological diseases other than idiopathic parkinsonism (Table 90.1). Most of these diseases are easily distinguished from idiopathic parkinsonism. However, the occurrence of otherwise typical parkinsonism and dystonia in children or young adults should prompt a workup for treatable etiologies, particularly Wilson's disease. The evaluation should include CT or MRI scans, serum copper and ceruloplasmin and slit-lamp examination to rule out Wilson's disease. If marked improvement in dystonia and parkinsonism occurs with small doses of levodopa, the patient may have 'dopa-responsive dystonia', an autosomal dominant disorder (with reduced penetrance). The syndrome begins in childhood or adolescence with dystonia and parkinsonism; the symptoms typically have diurnal fluctuations

Table 90.1   Diseases producing dystonia and parkinsonism

Idiopathic parkinsonism
Multiple system atrophy
Progressive supranuclear palsy
Vascular parkinsonism
Postencephalitic parkinsonism
Wilson's disease
Huntington's disease
Hallervorden–Spatz disease
Multiple sclerosis
Dopa-responsive dystonia and parkinsonism (Segawa syndrome)
Sporadic or familial basal ganglial calcification (Fahr's disease)
Hemiatrophy–hemiparkinsonism
Spinocerebellar degenerations

in severity. Rest alleviates the signs and exertion exacerbates them (Nygard *et al.*, 1991).

Treatment of coexisting dystonia and parkinsonism can be challenging. Dystonia, particularly of the lower extremities, may respond to levodopa. In other patients, the parkinsonism may improve with levodopa but the dystonia remains unaffected. Finally, in a significant proportion of patients, the levodopa improves the parkinsonism but worsens the dystonia. Levodopa combined with anticholinergics or dopamine agonists may offer better concurrent control of parkinsonism and dystonia (Klawans and Paleologos, 1986; LeWitt *et al.*, 1986; Poewe *et al.*, 1988). Bracing may be helpful for some limb dystonias and botulinum toxin injections can be used to ameliorate many dystonic syndromes (Jankovic and Brinn, 1991). For dystonia with contractures, orthopedic surgical treatment may be necessary.

91. *Akathisia may complicate Parkinson's disease*

Akathisia, a subjective restlessness and compulsion to move that is generally accompanied by objective restlessness, can occur in parkinsonism. The restlessness can take many forms; repetitive crossing and uncrossing the legs, readjusting body position while sitting, kicking, and pacing. The movements of akathisia are differentiated from levodopa-induced dyskinesia both by their normal character (rather than being choreoathetotic or dystonic) and by the patient's compulsion to move that is not caused by pain or other sensory symptoms which might cause restlessness. Akathisia must be differentiated from restlessness occurring in patients suffering pain from any cause including parkinsonism (see maxim 91), as well as from the restless legs syndrome, other sensory disturbances, stiffness and cramps. Agitation can also be confused with akathisia.

Although occasionally akathisia is so severe as to be disabling, the symptoms are rarely a major complaint. Akathisia is not rare; Lang and Johnson (1987) found that 26% of a nonselected group of patients with parkinsonism gave a history suggestive of akathisia and an additional 17% may have had very mild akathisia. The relationship of akathisia to parkinsonism or treatment is not clear. In some patients, akathisia may appear early in the course of the disease, before treatment is initiated. More commonly it occurs later, when the patient is receiving levodopa. Levodopa may reduce akathisia, may appear to cause it or may seemingly be unrelated to the symptom. Manipulation of dopaminergic drugs is rarely helpful. By analogy with neuroleptic induced-akathisia, propranolol may improve the symptoms; an anticholinergic is also worth a try.

92. *Sensory disturbances, particularly pain, may be the most disabling feature of the disease*

Although not widely recognized, pain and sensory symptoms are relatively common in parkinsonism; they require some attention to discern whether they are (1) an intrinsic non-motor aspect of the disease, (2) secondary to a motor manifestation of the disease, or (3) due to an unrelated condition.

A particular kind of primary parkinsonian pain that is especially distressing to the patient and puzzling to the physician is a poorly localized, deep, boring, tearing, burning pain, most commonly in the low back, buttocks, and legs, but sometimes affecting the abdomen, trunk or arms; this can be mistaken for angina or intra-abdominal pathology. It may be the first symptom of parkinsonism (maxim 10), but more often appears later in the course of the disease. Even late in the course of the disease, pain may overshadow the motor symptoms and present a major problem in clinical management.

> A 67-year-old man had the onset of a burning, aching pain in his buttocks and posterior thighs one year after the diagnosis of idiopathic parkinsonism. EMG and nerve conduction velocities were normal. Imaging of the lumbosacral spinal canal did not reveal root compression. The pain was his most disabling symptom, and he would 'overdose' on his Sinemet because the drug seemed to relieve his discomfort. Observation on the clinical research unit confirmed an 'off' pattern to the pain, which was present when the

Table 92.1 Pain and sensory symptoms

Primary symptoms	A. Pain
	1. aching
	2. deep, boring
	B. Paresthesia
	1. thermal (cold or burning)
	2. tingling, prickling
	C. Numbness
Secondary to motor manifestations	A. Aching secondary to rigidity and bradykinesia
	B. Pain associated with dyskinesia and dystonia
	C. Radiculopathy caused or exacerbated by dyskinesia
Associated musculoskeletal disorders	
	A. Frozen shoulder
	B. 'Shoulder–hand' syndrome
	C. Nocturnal cramp
Miscellaneous Intercurrent illness	Restless legs syndrome

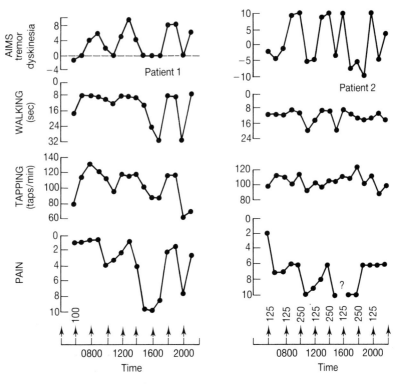

Fig. 92.1 Sensory Symptoms in Parkinsonism related to central dopaminergic function. (*Lancet* 1984; **2**: 456–7 (letter)). Pain is on a 0 = no pain to 10 = severe pain scale. Levodopa was administered at the times indicated by the arrows.

patient's parkinsonism was most prominent but would disappear when the levodopa was working and he was 'on'. A constant intravenous infusion of levodopa eliminated the pain for the duration of the infusion.

In this example the pain appeared during 'off' periods – the most common circumstance. In some patients, however, the pain fluctuates in a diphasic pattern just like the motor response (Quinn *et al.*, 1986). The pain may occur only when the levodopa begins to work or to wear off, and the pain disappears when the patient is either fully 'on' or fully 'off'.

The observation that the pain may fluctuate with the motor response to dopaminergic therapy and abate for the duration of an intravenous infusion of levodopa suggests that a disturbance in central dopaminergic function is in some way involved in the genesis of this pain (Nutt and Carter, 1984). The basal ganglia are known to receive and respond to sensory input; further newly discovered dopaminergic pathways projecting to thalamus and spinal cord could provide the anatomic connections which mediate a dopaminergic influence on pain perception.

The timing of the pains in relation to the levodopa dose and the appearance of the pain, in most patients, after years of therapy, suggests that the levodopa is in some way responsible for the pain. However, paradoxically most patients have less pain when they increase the dose, a technique which may be the best way to overcome the pain provided that a disabling increase in dyskinesias does not accompany the increased dosage. In a few patients the pain has been alleviated by total cessation of the drug; such is impractical in most patients (Quinn *et al.* 1986).

Pain also can be secondary to the motor abnormalities of the disease. Aching in the neck, back and shoulders is often secondary to rigidity and is relieved when drug treatment improves rigidity and mobility. It may also be caused by prolonged or severe dyskinesia of the neck. Cramping pain in the calf and/or foot may occur in association with dystonia of the foot and may be the first symptom of parkinsonism in a few patients. Painful 'off' dystonia is a complication of chronic levodopa therapy (see maxim 59). Most commonly flexion of the toes occurs, but hyperextension of the great toe ('striatal toe') may accompany painful inversion of the foot. Dystonic cramps are often precipitated by walking and may be mistaken for intermittent claudication.

Ordinary nocturnal cramps responsive to quinine seem to occur with greater frequency in parkinsonism. Sometimes they are associated with symptoms of restless legs. In severely symptomatic cases that respond poorly to dopaminergic therapy, drugs used for restless legs syndrome, such as codeine, benzodiazepines and valproate, may be tried. To reduce the considerable risk of side-effects in this elderly population, a small single nocturnal dose should be given.

Occasionally, limb pain from parkinsonism may have a radicular character and simulate either sciatica or cervical radiculopathy. One must also keep in mind, however, that a radiculopathy may be precipitated or aggravated by the cervical or truncal dyskinesia. Objective sensory findings or reflex changes are indicative of radiculopathy. If the pain responds to levodopa – a most important observation – the pain is the primary idiopathic pain of parkinsonism and is not caused by another disorder which requires further investigation.

93. *Falling is a multifactorial problem in elderly parkinsonian patients*

Falling is a common problem in the elderly and much more so in the elderly person with parkinsonism. Falling causes fractures and other medical complications, seriously limits mobility – and hence quality of life and independence – and often precipitates nursing home placement. It is thus an extremely important problem for the physician to address.

Falls in the elderly are complex because multiple factors often contribute.

Extrinsic risk factors for falls include environmental hazards like poor lighting, slippery or cluttered floors, walkways and stairs, bathrooms without grab bars and non-skid floors and bath surfaces, and crowded kitchens requiring reaching or climbing to obtain stored items. Inappropriate clothing, especially footwear, may contribute to falls. These problems can be assessed and corrective measures instituted during home visits by physical therapists and occupational therapists (Tinneti and Speechley, 1989).

Intrinsic risk factors for falls include: (1) sedative–hypnotic drug usage, (2) dementia, (3) orthostatic hypotension, (4) abnormalities of visual, vestibular and proprioceptive function, and (5) musculoskeletal disorders. The high correlation between sedative–hypnotics and falls requires a careful assessment of the value of these drugs in a patient's management and mandates attempts to reduce the use of these as well as other drugs in these patients (Tinneti and Speechley, 1988). Both poor judgement and inattention contribute to falls; these symptoms may respond to education of the patient and caregivers as well as to increased supervision. The approach to orthostatic hypotension is described in maxim 83.

In addition to the usual causes for falls seen in many elderly individuals, parkinsonism may cause falls by several additional mechanisms (Table 93.1). Optimization of antiparkinsonian medications is one major approach to avoiding falls attributable either to parkinsonism or to the medications. Shuffling may respond to increased dopaminergic stimulation. Freezing is peculiar; although it is sometimes caused by inadequate dopaminergic stimulation and will thus respond to an increase in levodopa, less commonly it may be caused by excessive dopaminergic stimulation and is improved by reduction of dopaminergic agents (Ambani and Van Woert, 1973). Unfortunately, freezing is often resistant to pharmacological manipulation. Likewise, impaired standing and postural reflexes are inconsistently affected by dopaminergic therapy, suggesting that these long-loop reflexes or responses are not solely under dopaminergic control.

The physician's or physical therapist's critical analysis of the postural responses, gait, and history of the falls can suggest other measures that may improve balance and gait (Table 93.2).

Table 93.1   Patterns of falls in parkinsonian patients

Tripping secondary to shuffling
Freezing and falling forward
Retropulsion leading to backwards falls
Disordered standing and protective reflexes leading to falls in any
    direction but particularly backwards and to the side
Dyskinesia interfering with standing or walking
Staggering and collapsing secondary to drug-induced orthostatic
    hypotension

Table 93.2   Techniques to improve balance and gait

Tripping	A. Avoid rubber and crepe shoe soles which catch on the floor; leather soles may be better
	B. Wear well-fitting, sturdy shoes
	C. Try ankle braces in patients who constantly 'catch their toe' and trip
	D. Experiment with canes and walkers
Freezing	A. Experiment with tricks to initiate gait, such as stepping over the handle of the inverted cane, trying to kick the cane, humming marching music, etc.
	B. Wear pads on knees and elbows and bicycle gloves to minimize injury from forward falls
	C. Instruct patient to walk slowly so that freezing will be less likely to cause a fall
Retropulsion	Use higher heels to keep center of mass forward and reduce retropulsion and backward falls
General considerations	A. Ensure that other neurological or medical problems are not contributing to balance and gait dysfunction
	B. Engage in strengthening, stretching and balancing exercise programs
	C. Educate regarding hazardous activities and safe ambulation
	D. Identify appropriate wheelchair or motorized carts for those unable to ambulate safely

94.   *Thalamotomy reduces controlateral rigidity, tremor and levodopa-induced dyskinesia*

Stereotactic surgery, introduced in 1946, was for 20 years the best treatment for parkinsonism. The targets of the stereotactic surgery were, initially, the globus pallidus interna and ansa lenticularis and, subsequently, the ventral lateral nucleus of the thalamus. Properly placed thalamic lesions reduced or abolished contralateral rigidity and tremor but had little effect on bradykinesia. The complications of unilateral surgery were dysarthria, dysphasia (for operations on the dominant thalamus), confusion, hemiparesis, sensory symptoms and involuntary movements. These adverse effects were generally mild and not of major consequence. Eventually parkinsonism becomes bilateral, necessitating a second operation on the other thalamus to control the symptoms. The second operation, unfortunately, was accompanied by more frequent and severe complications, particularly dysarthria and dysphagia, and surgeons became reluctant to perform bilateral operations. Furthermore, the outcome of the surgery was best in unilaterally affected patients or those with mild bilateral disease; more severely affected patients had a poorer outcome and more frequent complications. Thus the surgery was most successful in only a subset of patients with parkinsonism.

The introduction of levodopa in 1967 resulted in virtual abandonment of thalamotomy for the treatment of parkinsonism, especially because the drug relieved the bradykinesia as well as the rigidity and tremor and had no surgical complications. Nevertheless, there has been a rekindling of interest in neurosurgical treatment of parkinsonism because levodopa is not effective or not tolerated in all patients and because levodopa treatment is also not without complications. Furthermore, improvements in imaging with CT and MRI scanning and improvements in stereotactic guidance of the probes to specified targets should improve the accuracy of lesion placement and consequently the success of the operation. Chronic stimulation, rather than lesioning, of the thalamus has recently been shown to also be effective in treating tremor and rigidity with fewer permanent side-effects (Benabid *et al.*, 1991). Currently, indications for thalamotomy are: (1) severe, disabling tremor or rigidity, preferably unilateral and unaccompanied by marked bradykinesia that is unresponsive to drug therapy (Tasker *et al.*, 1983; Wester and Hauglie-Hansen, 1990); and (2) severe, disabling levodopa-induced dyskinesia, preferably unilateral, that limits the usefulness of levodopa therapy (Narabayashi *et al.*, 1984). Surgery is successful in reducing or abolishing contralateral tremor or levodopa-induced dyskinesia in 80% of patients undergoing the procedure. Mortality is virtually nil, and clinically significant, persistent morbidity was less than 10% in several recent series (Tasker *et al.*, 1983; Narabayashi *et al.*, 1984; Webster and Hauglie-Hansen, 1990). A successful thalamotomy for both of the indications above is described in the following case report.

> A 36-year-old woman had developed a resting tremor in her right hand at age 28. Levodopa was initiated a few years later with a good response. By age 34 she was experiencing a fluctuating response with intermittent, severe 'off' right hemidystonia and also peak-dose dystonia. Decreasing the size of each levodopa dose accentuated the frequency, severity and duration of the 'off' periods; increasing the levodopa increased the severity and duration of the 'on' dystonia. The dystonia abated with levodopa withdrawal, but anticholinergics and pergolide did not adequately control her severe right-sided tremor. Painful, 'off' dystonia recurred with reintroduction of levodopa. A left thalamotomy completely abolished the right-sided tremor and rigidity. She was managed without dopaminergic agents for two months until increasing hypophonia and gait disturbance necessitated reintroduction of small doses of levodopa and pergolide; these medications improved her parkinsonism without producing 'on' or 'off' dystonia.

A new potential target for stereotactic surgery, and a new manner in which to produce lesions, has been suggested by recent work in monkeys with MPTP-induced parkinsonism. Introduction of the neurotoxin, ibotenic acid, into the subthalamic nucleus, reduces tremor, rigidity and bradykinesia in the MPTP-lesioned monkey. Further studies are required to determine if this therapeutic lesion might be more effective than thalamotomy (Bergman *et al.*, 1990). Ibotenic acid does not affect fibers of passage but only cell bodies. The drug may therefore be associated with fewer complications than are induced by thermal or electrolytic lesions which destroy all tissue in the vicinity of the probe.

95. *General surgery can be complicated by drug interactions, neuroleptic malignant syndrome and delirium*

Surgery can usually be performed without undue risk in the parkinsonian patient, but the physician should be aware of potential problems.

Preoperative assessment should evaluate respiratory function. Patients may have restrictive pulmonary function (see maxim 84), abnormal cough, or inadequate control of oral secretions, all of which may be important in planning post-operative care.

Dopaminergic agents can potentially cause cardiac arrhythmias and hypotension. Arrhythmias have not emerged as a major problem, probably because combining a peripheral decarboxylase inhibitor with the levodopa reduces peripheral generation of dopamine; the latter mediates the arrhythmic effects by acting on the cardiac beta-adrenergic receptor (Ngai, 1972). Neither has hypotension been a major problem. For these reasons levodopa is generally stopped only the night before or even as little as four hours prior to surgery. The longer-lasting dopamine agonists are stopped the day prior to surgery. Selegiline is stopped several days prior to surgery even though the inhibition of MAO-B persists for weeks after cessation of the drug.

The drugs are restarted as soon after surgery as the patient can take medications by mouth. For patients who are NPO after major abdominal surgery, levodopa (Sinemet or Madopar) can be crushed and put down a nasogastric tube. If the suction on the tube is then turned off for 15–30 minutes, absorption of the drug should be adequate if it can enter the duodenum. Rectal administration of levodopa is ineffective. Parenteral forms of the anticholinergics (benztropine) may be used as well. Intravenous levodopa or apomorphine would be excellent for treating the post-operative patient, but neither are generally available. Dangers in not restarting the antiparkinsonian medications promptly include: patient discomfort, poor respiratory effort, poor cough, neuroleptic malignant syndrome and all the other complications which are associated with drug holidays (maxim 96).

Certain drugs should be avoided. Droperidol and antiemetics are dopaminergic antagonists which can worsen parkinsonism. Pethidine may interact with nonselective monoamine oxidase inhibitors to produce a neuroleptic malignant syndrome; this complication has recently been reported with selegiline as well (Zornberg *et al.*, 1991).

Delirium is particularly common in parkinsonian patients during the postoperative period (Golden *et al.*, 1989). Often there is a lucent period between the surgery and the delirium. The temptation to reduce the anti-parkinsonian drugs because they are a potential contributor to the delirium may lead to marked worsening of the parkinsonism. Frequently, a cause for the postoperative delirium cannot be identified in these patients (Golden *et al.*, 1989) although the physician should keep the differential for delirium in mind (maxim 75).

96. *Neuroleptic malignant syndrome is a potentially lethal complication of levodopa withdrawal*

Neuroleptic malignant syndrome is characterized by fever, autonomic instability, muscle rigidity and altered level of consciousness. Temperature can exceed 41°C autonomic signs include tachycardia, hypo- and hypertension and diaphoresis. The muscle rigidity is generally parkinsonian lead-pipe rigidity, although dystonia, chorea and opisthotonus have also been described. The rigidity is commonly associated with elevations of creatine kinase (CK) and occasionally with frank rhabdomyolysis and renal failure. The level of consciousness ranges from normal to coma, but more than three-quarters of the patients have some abnormality. The major medical complications of the syndrome are respiratory failure, renal failure and cardiovascular collapse (Guze and Baxter, 1985; Ebadi *et al.*, 1990; Keyser and Rodnitzky, 1991).

As evidenced by the name, the neuroleptic malignant syndrome is most commonly associated with administration of neuroleptics, generally to psychotic patients. However, the syndrome has been documented in patients with idiopathic parkinsonism, drug-induced parkinsonism, striatonigral degeneration, Wilson's disease and Huntington's disease. Furthermore, any pharmacologic manipulation capable of decreasing dopaminergic neurotransmission may precipitate the syndrome. Thus, withdrawal of levodopa, bromocriptine, amantadine and the anticholinergics or the addition of lithium or a neuroleptic to the drug regimen has caused the neuroleptic malignant syndrome in parkinsonian patients. The syndrome is also one complication of 'drug holidays' (see maxim 61). The interval between the alteration in the drug regimen and the appearance of the signs of the neuroleptic malignant syndrome ranges from one to nine days (Friedman *et al.*, 1985; Keyser and Rodnitzky, 1991).

The most important point about treatment is to recognize the syndrome promptly and to reinstitute or increase antiparkinsonian drugs and to withdraw neuroleptics or lithium. The differential for neuroleptic malignant syndrome includes infection (CNS, pulmonary, urinary, other), heat stroke, lethal catatonia, malignant hyperthermia associated with anesthesia, anticholinergic intoxication and drug interactions with nonselective monoamine oxidase inhibitors. Selegiline, a MAO-B inhibitor, appears to be largely free of these interactions, although an interaction with pethidine has been reported.

Treatment is directed to restoring dopaminergic neurotransmission by administration of antiparkinsonian medications such as levodopa, bromocriptine or amantadine. If the patient has recently been withdrawn from an anticholinergic, this type of agent should also be restarted. If rigidity is severe and unresponsive to the dopaminergic agents, intravenous dantrolene can be used to reduce the muscle rigidity. Aggressive medical management of pulmonary, renal and cardiac failure is required and infection must be excluded by appropriate evaluation. The neuroleptic malignant syndrome is associated with significant mortality that can be reduced by early diagnosis and prompt, aggressive treatment.

References

Ambani LM, Van Woert MH. Start hesitation – a side-effect of long-term levodopa therapy. *N Engl J Med* 1973; **288**: 1113–15.

Benabid AL, Pollak P, Gervashon C, *et al.* Long-term suppression of tremor by chronic stimulation of the ventral intermediate thalamic nucleus. *Lancet* 1991; **337**: 403–6.

Bergman H, Wichmann T, DeLong MR. Reversal of experimental parkinsonism by lesions of the subthalamic nucleus. *Science* 1990; **249**: 1436–38.

Bushmann M, Dobmeyer SM, Leeker L, Perlmutter JS. Swallowing abnormalities and their response to treatment in Parkinson's disease. *Neurology* 1989; **39**: 1309–14.

Critchley EMR. Speech disorders of parkinsonism: a review. *J Neurol Neurosurg Psych* 1981; **44**: 751–8.

Edwards LL, Pfeiffer RF, Quigley EMM, Hofman R, Balluff M. Gastrointestinal symptoms in Parkinson's disease. *Movement Dis* 1991; **6**: 151–6.

Ebadi M, Pfeiffer RF, Murrin LC. Pathogenesis and treatment of neuroleptic malignant syndrome. *Gen Pharmacol* 1990; **21**: 367–86.

Friedman JH, Feinberg SS, Feldman RG. A neuroleptic malignant-like syndrome due to levodopa therapy withdrawal. *JAMA* 1985; **254**: 2792–5.

Golden WE, Lavender RC, Metzer WS. Acute postoperative confusion and hallucinations in Parkinson's disease. *Ann Int Med* 1989; **111**: 218–22.

Guze BH, Baxter LR. Neuroleptic Malignant Syndrome. *N Engl J Med* 1985; **313**: 163–6.

Jankovic J, Brin MH. Drug therapy *N Engl J Med* 1991; **324**: 1186–94

Keyser DL, Rodnitzky RL. Neuroleptic malignant syndrome in Parkinson's disease after withdrawal or alteration of dopaminergic therapy. *Arch Inter Med* 1991; **151**: 794–6.

Klawans HL, Paleologos N. Dystonia–parkinson syndrome: differential effects of levodopa and dopamine agonists. *Clin Neuropharmacol* 1986; **9**: 298–302.

Kyriakides T, Hewer RL. Hand contractures in Parkinson's disease. *J Neurol Neurosurg Psychiat* 1988; **51**: 1221–3.

Lang AE, Johnson K. Akathisia in idiopathic Parkinson's disease. *Neurology* 1987; **37**: 477–81.

LeWitt PA, Burns RS, Newman RP. Dystonia in untreated parkinsonism. *Clin Neuropharmacol* 1986; **9**: 293–7.

Lipowski ZJ. Delirium in the elderly patient. *N Engl Med* 1989; **320**: 578–82.

Madrazo I, Drucker-Colin R, Diaz V, Martinez-Mata J, Torres C, Becerril JJ. Open microsurgical autograft of adrenal medulla to the right caudate nucleus in two patients with intractable Parkinson's disease. *N Engl J Med* 1987; **316**: 831–4.

Narabayashi H, Yokochi F, Nakajima Y. Levodopa-induced dyskinesia and thalamotomy. *J Neurol Neurosurg Psych* 1984; **47**: 831–9.

Ngai SH. Parkinsonism, levodopa and anesthesia. *Anesthesiology* 1972; **37**: 344–51.

Nutt JG, Carter JH. Sensory symptoms in parkinsonism related to central dopaminergic function. *Lancet* 1984; **II**, 456–7.

Nygaard TG, Marsden CD, Fahn S. Dopa-responsive dystonia: long-term treatment response and prognosis. *Neurology* 1991; **41**: 174–81.

Poewe WH, Lees AJ, Stern GM. Dystonia in Parkinson's disease: clinical and pharmacological features. *Ann Neurol* 1988; **23**: 73–8.

Purves-Stewart J. Paralysis agitans with an account of a new symptom. *Lancet* 1898; **2**: 1258–60.

Quinn N. Disproportionate antecollis in multiple system atrophy. *Lancet* 1989; **2**: 844.

Quinn NP, Lang AE, Koller WC, Marsden CD. Painful Parkinson's disease. *Lancet* 1986; **I**: 1366–9.

Quinn NP, Ring H, Honavar M, Marsden CD. Contractures of the extremities in parkinsonian subjects: a report of three cases with a possible association with bromocriptine treatment. *Clin Neuropharmacol* 1988; **11**: 268–77.

Rivest J, Quinn N, Marsden CD. Dystonia in Parkinson's disease, multiple system atrophy and progressive supranuclear palsy. *Neurology* 1990; **40**: 1571–8.

Severn AM. Parkinsonism and the anaesthetist. *Br J Anaesth* 1988; **61**: 761–70.

Tasker RR, Siqueira J, Hawrylyshyn P, Organ LW. What happened to VIM thalamotomy for Parkinson's disease? *Appl Neurohysiol* 1983; **46**: 68–83.

Tinetti ME, Speechley M. Prevention of falls among the elderly. *N Engl J Med* 1989; **320**: 1055–9.

Tinetti ME, Speechley M, Ginter SF. Risk factors for falls among elderly persons living in the community. *N Engl J Med* 1988; **319**: 1701–7.

Wester K, Hauglie-Hansen E. Stereotaxic thalamotomy – experiences from the levodopa era. *J Neurol Neurosurg Psych* 1990; **53**: 427–30.

Yorkston KM, Buekelman DR, Bell KR. *Clinical Management of Dysarthric Speakers.* Boston: Little Brown, 1988.

Zornberg GL, Bodkin JA, Cohen BM. Severe adverse interaction between pethidine and selegiline. *Lancet* 1991; **337**: 246.

15
Future Therapies

97. *Targeted and controlled delivery of drugs is the key to better symptomatic treatment of parkinsonism*

The three major themes in the development of better symptomatic therapies for parkinsonism are: (1) more specific agents, (2) better delivery systems, and (3) exploitation of neurotransmitter systems other than dopamine.

Many of the adverse effects of levodopa – such as nausea, orthostatic hypotension, hallucinations, and confusion – are presumed to reflect the action of dopamine either on different dopamine receptor subtypes or on dopamine receptors which are in different parts of the brain from those responsible for levodopa's beneficial effects. Thus, methods to target delivery of dopaminergic agents to the dopamine receptors of the basal ganglia – that are critical for normal movement – might avoid many unwanted dopaminergic effects. Progress in this direction is being made by the characterization of additional dopamine receptor subtypes and their anatomical localization. The preferential expression of the D3, D4 and D5 dopamine receptor subtypes in limbic structures suggests that the mental effects of dopaminergic stimulation may be mediated by these receptor subtypes (Sokoloff *et al.*, 1990; Van Tol *et al.*, 1991). Development of dopaminergic agonists with activity only at putaminal D1 and D2 receptor subtypes might then avoid adverse effects described above. Although such agonists are not currently available, a relatively specific D4 receptor subtype antagonist, clozapine, is available (Van Tol *et al.*, 1991). This atypical antipsychotic drug has virtually no extrapyramidal side-effects (Baldessarini and Frankenburg, 1991). More problematic is whether dyskinesia can be separated from the beneficial effects of dopaminergic stimulation; fortunately, there is some evidence for the pharmacologic differences between the dyskinesia and the antiparkinsonian effects (Boyce *et al.*, 1990).

The optimal temporal pattern for dopaminergic stimulation is not known. Because fluctuations in the clinical response of levodopa-treated patients correlate with fluctuations in plasma drug concentrations, one might assume that methods to maintain constant dopaminergic stimulation would reduce the 'wearing off' and the 'on–off'. Although, over the short run, this method is effective, we do not know if continuous dopaminergic stimulation is desirable, especially since tolerance may develop to dopaminergic agents (Cedarbaum *et al.*, 1990). Nevertheless, methods to prolong the action of each dose of levodopa would be helpful. Techniques include prolongation of the plasma half-life of levodopa by inhibiting its metabolism by catechol-o-methyl transferase or by the development of controlled-release preparations. Prolongation of the striatal half-life of dopamine by inhibition of monoamine oxidase or by inhibition of re-uptake may extend the clinical effects. The major thrust, however, is in 'delivery systems'. Among the technologies and procedures under investigation are implantable polymers which slowly release levodopa, systems of continuous direct delivery of drug into the duodenum through a PEG via mini pump, creation of blind loops of bowel for drug administration, and continuous subcutaneous administration of potent dopamine agonists by mini pumps.

The third major area of investigation for new symptomatic therapies is the manipulation of other basal ganglia neurotransmitter systems. Aside from dopamine, a number of other neurotransmitters and/or their synthesizing enzymes are altered in parkinsonism (Agid *et al.*, 1987), suggesting possibilities for pharmacological manipulation of these nondopaminergic systems which might improve parkinsonism. The system currently receiving the most interest is the glutaminergic projection from the subthalamic nucleus to the globus pallidus. Overactivity of this system appears to be related to parkinsonism, and reduction of the glutaminergic neurotransmission by lesioning the subthalamic nucleus or by antagonists of glutamate receptors improves MPTP-induced parkinsonism in monkeys (Bergman *et al.*, 1990; Brotchie *et al.*, 1991). As our understanding of basal ganglia neurotransmitter function grows, the possibility for therapeutic intervention increases.

98. *Development of preventive measures and protective therapies is dependent upon identifying risk factors for developing Parkinsonism and finding presymptomatic markers of the disorder*

The apparent success of selegiline in modifying the pathogenesis of parkinsonism (see maxims 32 and 38) has stimulated intense interest in other definitive therapies for parkinsonism. Identification of *the* causes of parkinsonism is obviously the key to developing better definitive treatment. However, the possibility that there is no single cause for idiopathic parkinsonism is being increasingly considered; instead, a multifactorial etiology – with genetic predisposition, age, and environmental toxins having roles – is considered more likely (see maxims 17 and 18). Potential environmental risk factors identified by studies include rural living, farming, drinking well-water and exposure to agricultural chemicals (Tanner and Langston, 1990). Endogenous risk factors identified by biochemical analysis of tissue include alterations in xenobiotic enzymes that metabolize exogenous chemicals, free radical protective mechanisms, and mitochondrial enzymes. Genetic studies complement these approaches since these enzymes are genetically determined. Risk factors may be present before the disease process begins (Fig. 98.1). Identification of risk factors is an important step to discovering the etiology(ies) of parkinsonism. Risk factors may identify subpopulations at risk for developing the disease for whom intervention with selegiline or other protective therapies would be beneficial (Langston and Koller, 1991).

A more modest research tactic is to seek markers of presymptomatic parkinsonism (Fig. 98.1) to delineate at-risk subpopulations for interventional therapies. A number of potential presymptomatic markers, including personality profiles, neuropsychological function, motor function, odor detection and electrophysiological tests, are under investigation

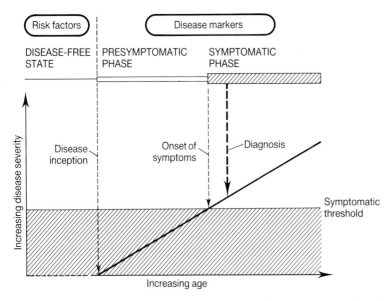

Fig. 98.1 Diagram illustrating presumed phases of development of parkinsonism: (1) a phase preceding the abnormal degeneration of dopaminergic neurons (*disease-free state*) only identifiable by risk factors; (2) a *presymptomatic phase* in which abnormal degeneration of dopaminergic neurons is occurring but without producing clinical signs (may be identifiable by biochemical or physiological tests of dopaminergic neurotransmission); and (3) a *symptomatic phase* when 80% of dopamine neurons have degenerated and signs and symptoms of parkinsonism are clinically evident. (Reproduced with permission from Langston and Koller, 1991)

(Langston, 1990). The problem with presymptomatic markers dependent upon function is that they are unlikely to be specific for parkinsonism. In the long history of searching for a presymptomatic marker for Huntington's disease – which employed all the above suggested markers – none was found to be specific enough to be a clinically useful marker. More promising are the biochemical markers of abnormalities of the dopaminergic system. Although positron emission tomography (PET) with fluorodopa can detect apparent presymptomatic parkinsonism by a decrease in fluorine retention in the striatum (Brooks, 1991), this technology is not suitable for screening large populations because it is very labor, time and cost intensive. Cerebrospinal fluid concentrations of dopamine precursors and metabolites, antibodies to dopamine neurons, and growth factors are being investigated as neurochemical indicators of presymptomatic or early disease.

The final common pathways for neuronal death may be similar for many diseases of the nervous system regardless of the initiating events. A role for free radicals in cell death is postulated for parkinsonism (maxim 38) as well as many other systemic diseases. Likewise, excitotoxicity, mediated by glutamate and glutamate receptors, is implicated in many neurologic disorders. Some evidence suggests that excitotoxicity plays a role in dopamine cell death as well (Sonsalla *et al.*, 1989; Taylor, 1991). Finally, alterations in calcium homeostasis are a common penultimate event in cell death (Schanne *et al.*, 1979). Possibilities for modifying any or all of these processes are under investigation; if they do contribute to dopaminergic neuron destruction, pharmacologic intervention may be possible.

99.　*Brain-grafting is a change in strategy from controlling symptoms to curing the disease*

If cells, releasing the appropriate neurotransmitters, could be grafted into the brain where they could establish functional contacts with denervated host neurons, permanent reversal of parkinsonism might be possible (Lindvall, 1989). The pathophysiology of idiopathic parkinsonism makes it an attractive candidate for brain grafting. The major symptoms of parkinsonism are the result of the degeneration of an anatomically well-defined set of neurons in the substantia nigra that release dopamine on to functionally intact striatal neurons. Furthermore, the substantia nigra tonically inhibits striatal neurons, and spatial and temporal coding of dopamine release is thereby believed to be unnecessary, thus explaining why dopaminergic drugs succeed in replacing the endogenous neurotransmitter. Some investigators have suggested that the donor tissue need act only as a 'mini-pump' for bathing the striatum with dopamine (Sladek and Gash, 1988). However, animal studies have demonstrated that the extent of synaptic contacts between the graft and host tissue are important in determining the success of the graft, as measured by the reversing of the deficits (Bjork-lund et al., 1987).

Two sources of tissue for brain grafting in idiopathic parkinsonism have been used: adrenal medullary autograft and fetal midbrain. The first approach was to graft the host's own adrenal medullary chromaffin cells into the striatum. Previous animal experiments had shown that in the striatum, the chromaffin cell releases dopamine rather than its usual neuro-hormone, noradrenalin. The first attempts using the stereotaxic placement of a cell suspension into the striatum resulted in no benefit to two patients. Because animal studies indicated that the chromaffin cells survived best in the ventricular system next to the caudate, an open surgical approach to implant pieces of adrenal medulla in the caudate in contact with ventricular CSF was attempted. The initial reports were extremely encouraging (Mad-razo et al., 1987), but with wider experience it became apparent that the dramatic results reported could not be duplicated. For most patients the morbidity of the procedure outweighed benefit (Lewin, 1988). The North American experience can be summarized as follows: approximately one-third of patients experience a measurable but modest improvement that diminishes with time, a third are no worse, and a third continue to worsen and/or suffer significant morbidity or mortality from the procedure (Goetz et al., 1991). Autopsies have shown that the grafted adrenal cells fail to survive (Waters et al., 1990). The favorable clinical response in a third of the patients is attributed to sprouting of surviving nigral nerve terminals stimulated by the procedure. This regenerative response is probably due to an increase in the local concentration of growth factors produced by the host brain in response to the grafting procedure and elaborated by the graft before it dies.

The second approach is the grafting of fetal midbrain which offers the theoretical advantage of providing nigral neurons that can differentiate and make synaptic contacts with the host striatum. In experimental animals this approach has proven to be superior to grafting chromaffin cells (Brun-din et al., 1988). Because of the difficulty in obtaining fetal tissue at the proper stage of development, ethical concerns, and the lack of US federal funding of research in this area, few patients have been treated. Fetal tissue grafts also require chronic immunosuppression. Thus far, results have been reported only in a handful of patients (Lindvall et al., 1990); judgements about the place of this approach in the treatment of idiopathic parkinson-ism are premature.

Finally, a novel source of donor tissue for brain grafting is cultured cells or tissues that can be genetically engineered to produce the appropriate neurotransmitters and growth factors. Because of their ability to survive and divide in vitro, many of these cell lines are derived from neoplasms, such as neuroblastoma. Methods are being devised to insert genes that will promote their differentiation and prevent their neoplastic growth.

100.   *Reparative therapy holds promise as a future approach to treatment*

Reparative therapy is the application of growth factors that prevent further degeneration and stimulate the function of surviving neurons. The first growth factor to be discovered, nerve growth factor (NGF), stimulates the growth of (1) sensory neurons derived from neural crest, (2) sympathetic neurons, and (3) cholinergic neurons (which might be of value in Alzheimer's disease), but has no effect on dopamine neurons. Recently, a protein related to NGF has been discovered, brain-derived neurotrophic factor (BDNF), which stimulates the growth of many types of neurons, including substantia nigra dopamine neurons (Knusel *et al.*, 1991). Not only does BDNF stimulate the growth of fetal dopamine neurons in culture, but it also reduces the loss of cultured neurons exposed to MPP, the toxic metabolite of MPTP (Hyman *et al.*, 1991) (see maxim 21). Thus, one might envision both the prevention of progression and the reversal of parkinsonism by the administration of BDNF. However, whether it will protect or stimulate the growth of adult dopaminergic neurons is unknown. BDNF does not cross the blood–brain barrier, and drug delivery will not be simple. However, intraventricular perfusion, osmotic blood – brain barrier disruption, or other innovative pharmaceutical or molecular biological techniques may allow delivery of BDNF or similar growth factors to the appropriate areas of brain (Olson *et al.*, 1991).

References

Agid Y, Javoy-Agid F, Ruberg M. Biochemistry of neurotransmitters in Parkinson's disease. In: Marsden CD and Fahn S (eds), *Movement Disorders 2*. London: Butterworth, 1987: 166–230.

Baldessarini RJ and Frankenburg FR. Clozapine: a novel antipsychotic agent. *N Engl J Med* 1991; **321**: 746–54.

Bergman H, Wichmann T, DeLong MR. Reversal of experimental parkinsonism by lesions of the subthalamic nucleus. *Science* 1990; **249**: 1436–8.

Bjorklund A, Lindvall O, Isacson O, Brudin P, Wictorin K, Strecker RE, Clarke DJ, Dunnett SB. Mechanisms of action of intracerebral neural implants: studies on nigral and striatal grafts to the lesioned striatum. *TINS* 1987; **10**: 509–16.

Boyce S, Rupniak NMJ, Steventon MJ, Iverson SD. Differential effects of D1 and D2 agonists in MPTP-treated primates: functional implications for Parkinson's disease. *Neurology* 1990; **40**: 927–33.

Brooks DJ. Detection of preclinical Parkinson's disease with PET. *Neurology* 1991; **41** (suppl 2): 24–7.

Brotchie JM, Mitchell IJ, Sambrook MA, Crossman AR. Alleviation of parkinsonism by antagonism of excitatory amino acid transmission in the medial segment of the globus pallidus in rat and primate. *Movement Dis* 1991; **6**: 133–8.

Brundin P, Strecker RF, Widner H, Clarke DJ, Nilsson OG, Astedt B, Lindvall O, Bjorklund A. Human fetal dopamine neurons grafted in a rat model of Parkinson's disease: immunological aspects, spontaneous and drug-induced behavior, and dopamine release. *Exp Brain Res* 1988; **70**: 192–208.

Cedarbaum JM, Silvestri M, Kutt H. Sustained enteral administration of levodopa increases and interrupted infusion decreases levodopa dose requirements. *Neurology* 1990; **40**: 995–7.

Goetz CG, Stebbins GT, Klawans HL, Koller WC, Grossman RG, Bakay RAE, Penn RD and the United Parkinson Foundation Neural Transplantation Registry. United Parkinson's Foundation Neurotransplantation Registry on adrenal medullary transplants: presurgical, and 1- and 2-year follow-up. *Neurology* 1991; **41**: 1719–22.

Hyman C, Hofer M, Barde Y-A, Juhasz M, Yancopoulos GD, Squinto SP, Lindsay RM. BDNF is a neurotrophic factor for dopaminergic neurons of the substantia nigra. *Nature* 1991; **350**: 230–2.

Knusel B, Winslow JW, Rosenthal A, Burton LE, Seid DP, Nikolics K, Hefti F. Promotion of central cholinergic and dopaminergic neuron differentiation by brain-derived neurotrophic factor but not neurotrophin:3. *Proc Natl Acad Sci* 1991; **88**: 961–5.

Koller WC, Langston JW (eds). Preclinical detection of Parkinson's disease. *Neurology* 1991; **41** (suppl 2): 1–92.

Langston JW. Predicting Parkinson's disease. *Neurology* 1990; **40** (suppl 3): 70–4.

Langston JW, Koller WC. The next frontier in Parkinson's disease: presymptomatic detection. *Neurology* 1991; **41** (suppl 2): 5–7.

Lewin R. Cloud over Parkinson's therapy. *Science* 1988; **240**: 390–2.

Lindvall, O. Transplantation into the human brain: present status and future possibilities. *J Neurol Neurosurg Psychiat* 1989; **52** (special suppl): 39–54.

Lindvall O, Brundin P, Widner H, Rehncrona S, Gustavii B, Frackowiak R, Leenders KL, Sawle G, Rothwell JC, Marsden CD, Bjorklund A. Grafts of fetal dopamine neurons survive and improve motor function in Parkinson's disease. *Science* 1990; **247**: 574–7.

Madrazo I, Drucker-Colin R, Diaz V, Martinez-Mata J, Torres C, Becerril JJ. Open microsurgical autograft of adrenal medulla to the right caudate nucleus in two patients with intractable Parkinson's disease. *N Engl J Med* 1987; **316**: 831–4.

Olson L, Backlund E-O, Ebendal T, Freedman R, Hamberger B, Hansson P, Hoffer B, Lindblom U, Meyerson B, Stromberg I, Sydow O, Seiger A. Intraputaminal infusion of nerve growth factor to support adrenal medullary autografts in Parkinson's disease. *Arch Neurol* 1991; **48**: 373–81.

Quinn NP, Lang AE, Koller WC, Marsden CD. Painful Parkinson's disease. *Lancet* 1986; **I**: 1366–9.

Schanne FAX, Kane AB, Young EE, Farber JL. Calcium dependence of toxic cell death: a final common pathway. *Science* 1979; **206**: 700–2.

Sladek JR, Gash DM. Nerve-cell grafting in Parkinson's disease. *J Neurosurg* 1988; **68**: 337–51.

Sokoloff P, Giros B, Martres MP, Bouthenet ML, Schwartz JC. Molecular cloning and characterization of a novel dopamine receptor (D3) as a target for neuroleptics. *Nature* 1990; **347**: 146–50.

Sunahara RK, Guan HC, O'Dowd BF, *et al.* Cloning of the gene for a human D5 receptor with higher affinity for dopamine than D1. *Nature* 1991; **350**: 614–19.

Sonsalla PK, Nicklas WJ, Heeikkila RE. Role for excitatory amino acids in methamphetamine-induced nigrostriatal dopaminergic toxicity. *Science* 1989; **243**: 398–400.

Tanner CM, Langston JW. Do environmental toxins cause Parkinson's disease? A critical review. *Neurology* 1990; **40** (suppl 3): 17–30.

Taylor R. A lot of 'excitement' about neurodegeneration. *Science* 1991; **252**: 1380–1.

Van Tol HHM, Bunzow JR, Guan HC, *et al.* Cloning of the gene for a human dopamine D4 receptor with high affinity for the antipsychotic clozapine. *Nature* 1991; **350**: 610–14.

Waters C, Itabashi HH, Apuzzo MLJ, Weiner LP. Adrenal to caudate transplantation – postmortem study. *Movement Dis* 1990; **5**: 248–50.

Appendix 1
Lay Organizations

A number of lay organizations offer patient-oriented booklets, newsletters, audiovisual materials and information on clinical trials and local support groups.

Parkinson's disease

American Parkinson Disease Association (APDA), 60 Bay Street, Suite 401, Staten Island, NY 10301, USA
TEL: (800) 223–2732 or (718) 981–8001; FAX: (718) 981–4399

National Parkinson Foundation (NPF), 1501 NW 9th Avenue, Bob Hope Road, Miami, FL 33136, USA
TEL: (800) 327–4545 or (800) 433–7022 (Florida)

Parkinson's Disease Foundation (PDF), William Black Medical Building, 640 West 168th Street, New York, NY 10032, USA
TEL: (212) 923–4700

Parkinson's Educational Program (PEP), 3900 Birch Street Suite 105, Newport Beach, CA 92660, USA
TEL: (714) 640–0218

United Parkinson Foundation (UPF), 360 West Superior Street, Chicago, IL 60610, USA
TEL: (312) 664–2344

The Parkinson Foundation of Canada, Suite 232, ManuLife Centre, 55 Bloor Street West, Toronto, Ontario, M4W 1A6 Canada

Parkinson's Disease Society (of the United Kingdom), 22 Upper Woburn Place, London WC1H ORA, UK
TEL: 071–383-3513; FAX: 071–383-5754

Progressive supranuclear palsy

Society for Progressive Supranuclear Palsy (SPSP), c/o David Saks, 2904-B Marnat Road, Baltimore, MD 21209, USA

Appendix 2
Books for Patients with Parkinson's Disease and their Families

---

Caring for the Parkinson Patient (1989)
Editors: J Thomas Hutton and Raye Dippel
Publisher: Promethius Books, 700 East Amhurst, Buffalo, NY 14215, USA

Parkinson's Disease. . . One Step at a Time (1989)
Author: J David Grimes (MD), Peggy A Gray and Kelly A Grimes
Publisher: Parkinson's Society of Ottawa, Carleton Ottawa Civic Hospital,
1053 Carling Avenue, Ottawa, Ontario, K1Y 4E9 Canada

The Parkinson's Handbook
Author: Dwight C McGoon
Publisher: WW Norton & Co., New York, NY, USA

Parkinson's Disease: A Guide for Patient and Family (3rd edn, 1991)
Author: Roger C Duvoisin (MD)
Publisher: Raven Press, 1140 Avenue of the Americas, NY, NY 10036, USA

Parkinson's: A Patient's View
Author: Sidney Dorros
Publisher: Seven Locks Press, PO Box 72, Cabin John, MD, USA

We Are Not Alone: Learning to Live with Chronic Illness
Author: Sefra Pitzele
Publisher: Thompson Company Inc., Minneapolis, MN, USA

Living Well With Parkinson's: An Inspirational, Informative Guide for Parkinsonians and their Loved Ones
Authors: Glenda W Atwood and Lila G Hunnewell
Publisher: John Wiley and Sons

Index